*Aging with Joy* is both the name of a book and a description of an effective philosophy about people who want to enjoy their lives to the fullest. Again we meet an aged truth. It is not only what happens to us, but how we meet it that is the important issue. When a book makes me twinkle inside, I know it is a good one. This is the effect on me of *Aging with Joy*.

*Virginia Satir, ACSW*
*Director of Training,*
*AVANTA Network*

After the age of 20, the marking of each new decade in one's life brings its own feelings of mortality and aging. After 50 these may be supplemented with thoughts about what might have been, reflections on personal failures and regrets about relationships gone wrong. Loneliness and depression may even be new companions. And then there is the simple fact that sickness and pain enter your life even more frequently.

*Aging with Joy*, by Ruth Morrison and Dawn Dridan Radtke, offers good and sensible advice about how to cope with these elements and how to discover peace and happiness while growing older.

*Norman Perry, OFM*
*St. Anthony Messenger*

This book holds great promise for those who choose to age with joy. Each chapter reveals that self-determination and choice remain essential aspects of all phases of life. We indeed shape our lives.

Morrison and Radtke have a sound philosophical understanding of the human person based on the integration of spiritual, emotional, psychological, and physical components of life. They recognize the psychological and physical dimensions inherent in the aging process, and provide readers with action plans to shape, enrich, and enjoy the aging years.

*Teresa Houlihan, OP, PhD*
*Providence College*

||||||||||||||||||||||||||||||||||||||||||||||||||||||||||||||||||||||||||||||||||||||||||||||||||||||||||||||||||||||

I have read *Aging with Joy* several times and loved it better each time. What I like is that the authors address themselves to the elderly directly with very useful advice for living out their experiences usefully and joyfully.

My own philosophy about old age is that it can be the best time of life, if lived fully and creatively. The authors bring this to a very powerful conviction with thoughtful advice. For example, their treatment of loneliness is that it is not a problem but a challenge. I certainly gained much by reading this book.

*Louis J. Putz, CSC*
*Director, Forever Learning Institute*

||||||||||||||||||||||||||||||||||||||||||||||||||||||||||||||||||||||||||||||||||||||||||||||||||||||||||||||||||||||

*Aging with Joy* is a joy, a book long-awaited, and one that should be available for all Third Agers. Healthy, active retirees will find multiple suggestions for creating a new life; the frail elderly are offered ways to round out a long lifespan with dignity and a sense of completeness. All will find hope and new meaning.

For those working with the elderly, *Aging with Joy* offers insights and practical approaches to the many problems confronting those growing old in our society.

*Suzanne Kelly, PhD*
*Director, Programs for Church Leaders*
*University of Notre Dame*

||||||||||||||||||||||||||||||||||||||||||||||||||||||||||||||||||||||||||||||||||||||||||||||||||||||||||||||||||||||

I have worked clinically with elders who were having difficulty dealing with the many changes inherent in aging. I often wished for an adequate guidebook to help these people in understanding both the normal process of change and how to make aging a positive, growing experience. *Aging with Joy* fills this gap in a most exemplary way. It provides a pragmatic, problem-solving approach to very genuine problems, and it is a pleasure to read.

Morrison and Radtke not only dispel the stereotypes and myths of aging but they also show how the real changes of age can be understood and dealt with.

*Josie Wilson, PhD*
*Southern Oregon State College*

||||||||||||||||||||||||||||||||||||||||||||||||||||||||||||||||||||||||||||||||||||||||||||||||||||||||||||||||||||||

# AGING

## WITH

# *JOY*

### Ruth Morrison
### Dawn Dridan Radtke

## TWENTY-THIRD PUBLICATIONS
**Mystic, Connecticut**

Twenty-Third Publications
185 Willow Street
P.O. Box 180
Mystic, CT 06355
(203) 536–2611

ISBN 0-89622-360-4
Library of Congress Catalog Card Number 87-51567

Editing by Eleanor Buehrig
Cover design by Marianne Meyer

# ACKNOWLEDGMENTS

We want to thank five people who generously took their time to read our manuscript and who gave us their help to make this book more useful to its readers.

Lee Lester
Mooie Slater, M.S.S.W.
Sister Susan Marie, V.H.M.
Dorothy Vergeer, M.A.
Josie Wilson, Ph.D.

# CONTENTS

# Introduction

Aging is something we all share. We grow older each moment of our lives from birth to death. Our only choice is how we decide to live the days of our years. Some people simply endure the aging process. They bear with stoicism the changes and chances of growing older. Others, even though they are aware of their aging faces, their weakening physical bodies, and their diminishing mental capacities, manage to continue to like themselves, make new friends, and live with love, laughter, peace, and joy.

As the writers of this book have talked with men and women from middle age to old age, we have found that the only difference between the "endurers" and those who live with joy has been the attitude each has in facing the business of living. We have spoken and written to people of various educational backgrounds, economic circumstances, marital status, and cultural opportunities. In all groups, we have found "endurers" and those whose lives were filled with joy.

Looking at other books on aging, we found a great deal written about specific issues, but almost nothing written about how to stop "enduring" the aging years and start enjoying life.

It is of course much easier to talk about what's wrong than it is to suggest what will help. It is easier to point out negative patterns than it is to suggest ways for positive movement. We were not surprised, then, to find so little written about aging gracefully, aging with a sense of well-being—aging with joy.

We decided that a technical book with erudite quotations and findings from extensive research was not going to be helpful to most people. We chose rather to write out of our experience of talking with many people who have aged, projecting our own personal journeys into aging, and conducting workshops on aging throughout the United States.

As we begin to think about aging with joy, we realize that the aging process is another of life's many changes. Throughout the seasons and years of our life there are constant changes— beginnings and endings, comings and goings, anticipations and actualities.

During the first half of life the major emphasis is on growth, preparation, and hard work. While we live day to day we are getting ready to do anticipated things later. We learn letters so we will be able to read; read so we can accumulate more information and pass into the next grade in school; work hard to get the right education to prepare us for our chosen trade or profession so we can get the desired job. Once we have the job, we continue to strive for promotions, job security, and stability.

Simultaneously, we learn how to behave so we will please our parents and be accepted in our social situation; meet the right people and feel wanted and accepted; find the right partner to start our own family and give our children opportunities we never had.

For most of us, major changes take place somewhere around the forties, when many of our goals have been met and others have been altered. Often people change jobs, enter new professions or re-enter the workplace, set up a new set of goals and once again work hard to achieve them.

Concurrently, many prepare for retirement by setting aside resources or establishing IRAs, Keoughs, and other financial retirement plans. At the same time they begin to anticipate all they will be able to do with the extra time when they retire.

Somewhere in the sixties, many of these things for which we have been working become a present reality. We stop going to our working place. We no longer look ahead to the time we will have leisure. The time is now. It is right here. This is an exciting moment for us.

Unfortunately for many people, what should be fun and exciting is bewildering and frightening. They have had almost no preparation for this moment. Our culture has focused on helping prepare us for the next thing to do, but it has almost ignored how to close the door on our work world and many other things which have occupied our time until retirement. We need help as we face the tomorrows that become today.

This book concerns itself with issues of the now. It contains practical guidelines for you to follow so that your aging will not be simply endured, but will be lived with genuine joy. No one ever chooses to grow older, but unless we die before mid-life we do grow older and are sooner or later confronted by the facts of an aging life. We cannot alter the facts of change, aging, loss, pain, or death, but we can decide whether we will face those facts with anger, fear, and despair or with challenge, good humor, and joy.

The concept of joy is little understood in our day. In our Western culture we talk a lot about happiness and having a good time—and that usually means having a satisfying number of things which, for us, make for happiness. Advertisements usually entice us into believing that beauty products, clothes, automobiles, homes, televisions, VCRs, and travel guarantee happiness. More subtle are the goals we set for ourselves: education, employment, family, relationships, and community respect. These we believe will bring happiness.

Joy, however, is not related to any material possessions or achievements in education or work; nor is it dependent on what anyone else thinks of us. Joy is an inner state of being that comes from knowing that we are in tune with the universe, at one with ourselves, in good relationship with other people, and believe in a power beyond ourselves—God.

One of the best known persons of joy in our time is Mother Teresa, who lives in abject poverty among the poorest of India, but who lives with joy as she and her sisters share God's love with the men, women, and children who are called untouchables, the bottom of the Indian caste system.

Joy is what we see on the face of a little child, happy to be alive in this world of miracles, open to laughter, open to love.

Joy is what we see in the faces of a young man and woman as they leave the altar following the marriage ceremony to begin their lives together. Joy is what we see in the face of the mother as she holds her firstborn child in her arms and knows that she has been given a great gift from the Giver of life.

Joy is what we see in some of the very old who, having lived modest and quite simple lives, are now at peace as they live in their final years. Age we must. Age with joy, we may. We have written our book to help you age with true joy.

# Chapter 1

# Life Review

As we listen to people who have retired and who are not feeling comfortable about themselves, we hear expressions such as "I don't fit any more," "I'm nothing but a burden," "I'm not pulling my weight," "I don't want to spend time with all those old folks; they're such a drag," "There's no purpose to my life anymore," and "I wonder why I was born."

One of the activities which has proven useful to many in their later years is called the "life review." The process was developed and introduced by Robert N. Butler, M.D., who became the first director of the National Institute on Aging. As its name applies, it involves telling your own life story.

Some people, still able to do so, write their own story. Sometimes a friend or family member acts as a scribe or resource person. Some have chosen to illustrate their story with photographs, clippings, and the like, and a few have made their story with video equipment or tape recorders.

Suppose you choose to write your life story. Get yourself an attractively bound book of blank pages, give it a title, and go ahead. Decide what day you will start and how often you will do some work on it. For example, you may decide to start it next Wednesday and to give it some priority time each Wednesday until it is completed. Or you may decide to write for a set period of time—three or four times each week.

Start at the beginning and write what you know or imagine about the preparations for your birth, about you as an infant, and up through the years. Recall and write about such things as taking care of a pet, being big enough to go to the store alone and run errands for your mother, your first day at school, cheering at a ball game. You may remember learning to fish, to wash your own hair, or to drive. Getting your first job, going on a trip, your first date, having a child, or anything else you recall will be appropriate material.

This is your life's story. By all means mention other people and how they helped or hindered you, were kind or cruel; but always return to focus on your own actions, thoughts, and feelings, and allow the story to emerge and develop. As you proceed, you may have surprises as you recall your joys and sorrows, your peaks and valleys.

Your story will remind you of your uniqueness, your accomplishments, and your ability to live through whatever the circumstances were. You will be reminded of the many things you learned, the creative ideas you had, and the contributions you made.

As you ponder your life story, you will see how often you made a difference in your world when you "gooed" for your mother, learned to skip rope, carried a package for a lady, baked cookies for a neighbor, nurtured a child, had a kind word for a friend, taught a class of children, worked on a committee, helped someone in need, ran for political office, or did a good job for your boss—you did make a difference in your world.

As you do your review, you will also recall the rough times you had, the burdens, disappointments, sorrows, and tragedies you bore. No matter how troublesome or serious these were, you found a way to live through them and to endure. As you look back, you may well be amazed at the strength you were able to muster to live through severe troubles. Acknowledge the strength you had. If you are aware of carrying grudges and resentments, the next chapter will provide some ways for you to unload them.

The "life review" is yours and for you; however, if you want it to, it can also provide a legacy for your family and friends. It can provide something to give to those you love and care about.

Once you remind yourself and acknowledge that your family, your school, your friends, your company, and your town have been influenced, changed, or enhanced by you, do something concrete to help yourself take ownership of your unique contribution to this world. No other person has made, or could make, a similar contribution in quite the same way you did.

You can be as creative as you choose how you make this acknowledgment. Some things others do include the following:

1) Make a certificate or plaque of achievement.

2) Write a letter of appreciation to yourself.

3) Ask a friend or relative to write a letter of appreciation for you.

4) Think of something that symbolizes who you are or what you have done, and either make or buy something you can wear to remind you of that every day. For example, a man who was an ardent lover of nature and who worked hard to support his family, chose a maple tree as his symbol. He had a belt buckle made with a maple engraved upon it. Daily, it reminded him of his steadfastness in providing beauty, dignity, stability, and shelter for himself and his family, fuel to kindle warmth in the cold and dark times, shade in the summers, and food for their sustenance.

A woman chose a rose, which reminded her of her gentleness and sweetness as well as her assertiveness and her willingness to be a thorn when she needed to fight for her independence. For some time she searched for the right rose, and then had it made into a pendant.

Choose your symbol with care, wear it well, and if you prefer, keep the symbolic meaning a secret just for yourself.

Right now, concentrate only upon the constructive, loving, creative, joyful things you have done and the fine person you are. However, if old guilts or resentments get in your way, make a note of them until you get to Chapter 2.

In the introduction, we wrote of the disproportionate amount of time and energy we put into preparing for the future, in comparison with enjoying the present. Part of this enjoyment of the present is that when we do something—small or big—so often we immediately think, "Now what?"

Often what we do seems significant only when it is a stepping stone to something else that appears bigger, grander, or more noteworthy. This is a tragedy. It prevents us from finding joy in little things. It diminishes the value of much that we do and have done, and discourages taking pleasure in what we are doing today for today, or what we did last week or years ago for our yesterdays.

On the day you were born, you were given your birthright to be in this world. You were enough, simply because you were you. You did not need to do anything other than to be. As you grew and learned to do things, you may also have acquired the idea that you are "all right" only when you are doing something. That is not true. It is wonderful to be able to do things and to do them well; however, you have the right to be, simply because you are.

Having done your "life review," remind yourself that that was, and that you are enough for you. You do not need to do more to be or to stay "all right." You may choose to do more, but choosing because you want to, and are in a position to do so, is quite different from convincing yourself that you are "no good" unless you keep on doing more and more. You are enough.

# Chapter 2

# The Healing of Memories

Our painful memories often lie just below a thin layer of forgetfulness. Suddenly a seemingly small event can rip away that layer. We are again bruised, hurt, and bewildered. We had thought a painful memory was gone.

What has gone wrong is that we pushed away our earlier pain too quickly. We tried to be strong too soon. We need to look more deeply at how memories are healed. This chapter provides a way to heal our painful memories. Let us see how it all works.

We see a movie, read a book, look at television, sit in a restaurant, or walk along a street, and without any warning, we find ourselves very angry, trembling with fear, or crying, deep inside or sometimes with pitiful outer tears. We are surprised to feel what we feel. Only after a moment of reflection do we realize we have just seen someone who reminds us of a person who angered or frightened us, or who went away from us many years ago. We have, then, so to speak, opened an earlier unhealed wound with what seemed a very minor present happening.

If when we relive the present hurt, anger, fear, or sadness we continue to push it away again, calling ourselves stupid or childish, we miss the very thing that could lead us on to final healing. Every physician knows that wounds heal from their innermost depth outward to their surface. If the wound is covered over too quickly, it may fester and fill with pus, thereby creating great danger in our bodies. So it is with wounds of the heart and soul. Too early covering over anger, fear, and sadness will fester and fill us with the poison of infection. Some physical symptoms are simply the result of such poison (aching in head, neck, shoulders, back; skin eruptions, gastro-intestinal disturbances; respiratory difficulties; enervation). Some physicians believe that almost all physical symptoms have psychological origins and that if the emotional conditions are cleared the symptoms will disappear. If the emotional condition has lasted a long enough time, of course permanent organic damage may have been done. Such damage may cause severe pain, and medication or surgery may be needed, but much physical suffering will be relieved and disappear as our emotional well- being is restored. Chapter 7 elaborates on the relationship between body and mind, but in the meantime we do need to keep this relationship in our thinking as we speak about the healing of memories.

There are six steps that help in the healing of memories: (1) recall the memory; (2) relive the memory; (3) express the feeling that you had originally; (4) put a positive feeling in place of the hurtful one; (5) pray for God's healing; and (6) forget the pain and get on with the joy.

1) Recall. We have just spoken of the spontaneous recall triggered by some seemingly unrelated present event. What we are suggesting now is *planned* recall, that is, deliberately thinking about an unhealed wound which we now bring to our mind. An unhealed wound means a wound surrounded with large amounts of anger, sadness, or fear—memories that seem to take charge of us and destroy our tranquility and sense of joy of living. In recall, it is important to be completely honest rather than to push away and pretend to be mature and beyond our wound.

2) Relive. Once we are in touch with a specific unhealed wound, we are then ready to relive it. Reliving means to imagine ourselves back in time to that scene that was originally so painful for us. Imagine who was there, where everyone stood or sat, what the place looked like, who said and did what, and what we were experiencing. Then as the

old feelings come back (sadness, anger, fear) we are ready for the next step.

3) Express feelings. Express the feelings we then had in the present moment. Here it is important to realize that we will not be hurting anyone else if in private we express how we truly felt about them, whether it was anger, fear or sadness. If we were angry, we can now take a pillow, pretending it is the one who angered us, and we can literally hit that pillow to dispel our rage. We can draw a picture that depicts our anger or hurt or fear. We can write a letter (which we never send) that tells our feelings. Some people like to make clay figures to depict emotions. Whatever mode of expression we choose, it is important to keep expressing the feeling until the feeling is resolved. With anger, it is always good to use physical force such as hitting and to use our voices to make noise, since anger is part of the small child within us and anger carries with it a vast amount of negative energy. As we hit, yell, and throw, we are discharging this negative energy so that we can then fill ourselves with vital life-giving positive energy. The same principle applies to sadness and the importance of crying—the release of negative energy and the taking in of positive energy. When we have expressed our feelings often enough and made a conscious decision to let the negative feelings go, then we are ready to move on to step four.

4) Replace the negativity. Ask yourself, "What would I rather be than 'mad, sad, scared,' etc.?" Sometimes people have held on to so much anger, sadness, or fear for so many years that it takes quite a lot of self-searching to know what they would like to feel instead of these painful feelings. That self-searching will bring its own reward, however. When we give up an old habit, it is essential that we replace it with something else. Otherwise, what we do not want will fill the void. Jesus told the story of the man who swept his house clean of a devil, only to find several

other devils had come in by the back door, so to speak, and Jesus says the second state of that man was worse than the first. In place of a negative habit pattern another negative pattern hops in. To avoid this, one needs to decide what to slip in as the old is moving out. The following examples illustrate:

a) Instead of being "mad" at Mary, I will talk to her and see how we can be better friends.

b) Instead of feeling scared to get up before a group of people, I will accept a task of making an announcement to a small group, and gradually learn how to be comfortable when speaking in front of larger groups.

c) Instead of being sad that my mother did not seem to want me, I will learn to take good care of myself and be an inner mother to the little child within me.

In this new way of living with memories and seeking healing, this next step seeks outside help.

5) Pray. Many people today say that they find prayer meaningless, or that they do not know how to pray, or that they are confused in the matter of prayer. Problems such as these usually stem from rejection of childhood religious teaching which has not stood up under the realities of a person's life. This is not the place for a detailed exploration of theological issues concerning prayer. Suffice it to say that in working through the healing of memories as well as the other issues in this book, many will find that a power beyond their own is giving them added support and strength. A very simple way to think of prayer is to think about getting in touch with a power beyond our own and asking that power to uphold us and give us courage to live our lives without being defeated by negative thoughts and feelings. Prayer helps us fill ourselves with peace and joy, laughter, and love. St. Paul lists the gifts of God's Holy Spirit as "love, joy, peace, long-suffering, gentleness, goodness, faith, meekness, temperance." If I simply ask for

these gifts, I am told they will be given. As these gifts are given and as I accept them, painful memories are healed and life is more meaningful.

6) Forget. This is the final test in the healing of memories. Of course hurt, sadness, fear, and anger are forever a part of the human experience. To lose our ability to feel these things would be to lose part of our humanness, just as to lose love, tenderness, joy, and merry-making would be to become less than human. This final step of forgetfulness is to decide we will not give our energy to past wounds but instead commit ourselves to the love and joy of living this moment.

# Chapter 3

# Listening Partners

A *New Yorker* cartoon shows a little creature from outer space standing in the Arizona desert calling out, "Can anyone hear me?" His call is our call. We listen eagerly for an answer.

In our younger years we spent a good deal of time and energy being sure we were heard. At first we had only our baby cries to make our needs known. Later we used words to speak to playmates, family, neighbors, and friends. We called out and were heard and other people responded. Had we not been heard, we would not have survived.

In a classic study, Dr. Margaret Ribble of Columbia University discovered that infants die if they have their physical needs met but are not given enough touching, cuddling, and love. In another study, Dr. Renee Spitz discovered that if human beings did not get significant recognition from others, their spines quite literally shriveled and they became increasingly withdrawn from relationships. The poet John Donne wrote, "No man is an island, entire of itself." Sociologists, psychologists, and theologians tell us how necessary it is that we belong, that we relate in meaningful ways to others and that we care for them and are cared about.

As we grew older, we were probably separated from those who had been part of our caring group. Family and friends often moved away. Others became too aged to give us what they once did. Still others died and left our hearts empty as we longed for the closeness we once shared. Much as we understand that moving, sickness, aging and death are facts of life, we still need to be close and we still need to share love and care. It is not good to think that anyone can replace another and be to us what someone dear to us has been. Likewise, it is not good to hurt ourselves by not having new relationships of a close kind. Finding a listening partner can be a way of finding closeness.

A listening partner is a person who will agree to exchange time with you at fairly regular intervals (daily, weekly, or every other week). You should agree on the length of time for each of you to listen to the other in equal amounts—five minutes, fifteen—whatever time you both need. Find a family member, a friend or a would-be friend, who will agree to become a partner with you.

The time you spend together as partners should be divided into two parts: (1) What's wrong? and (2) What's good? Person A takes the agreed upon length of time to tell Person B everything that *is* wrong, negative, bad, sad, or disappointing about the time since they last talked together. When A has finished, B tells A about his or her bad times. In the second time period, divided equally between the two, each tells the other what's been good, fun, exciting, or happy. This means the exercise always ends on a positive note. Even if step one has been very painful and the world seems terrible, you can end on a happy note of thanksgiving that you have each other and for the caring you share with one another.

Any amount of time and any length of interval between sessions is fine, so long as you both agree and so long as you give equal time to each partner so that a system of genuine exchange occurs. Otherwise one may feel overburdened or undernourished. A word of caution: If, as you listen, your partner has deep pain and suffering, and repeats the same thing many times, you may begin to feel burdened and helpless. If your partner needs more than a listening ear, he or she may need professional help. In this special area, you may want to suggest seeking that help from a minister, priest, rabbi, counselor, or psychothera-pist. The two of you should then confine yourselves to other areas.

We have suggested this idea of listening partners to many people, especially to those who feel cut off and those who are living alone. Many people tell us how much these listening partnerships mean. Talking with others about current events, movies, television programs, and grand-children can pass time pleasantly. But we all need to share at a deeper level, our pains and our joys. "Listening part-ners" may be a way for you to be a friend and have a friend with whom you can do this deeper sharing.

# Chapter 4

# Live and Learn
# All Your Life

Are you living? What a strange question! You say, of course I'm alive or I would not be reading this book. Let us ask the question another way: Are you living or are you simply alive?

To be alive is to have living cells within our bodies. But to be alive is not the same thing as living. We are all alive in the cellular, biological sense but some of us have decided to die in the emotional, psychological and/or spiritual aspects of our being. There are people aged twenty, forty-three, sixty-one...who seem dead. Technically, they are alive, but the warm, feeling, growing human being seems no longer there.

What accounts for these deaths? Early psychical damage, lack of nurture, insufficient stimulation, negative associations and learning experiences, unassimilated traumatic events—these and many other factors stop learning and living. If you have stopped living and learning, if your life is often listless, if you would describe yourself as helpless, hopeless, and loveless, then we would like you to know that whatever your age, right now you can make a decision to start living again. Dr. Eric Berne, a California psychiatrist who began what came to be known as T.A. (Transactional Analysis), discovered that we make our major life decisions by the time we are six years old, eight at the latest. These decisions are lifelong unless they are consciously changed and new decisions are made. Happiness or unhappiness, success or failure, love or lovelessness, self-esteem or self-debasement—these are the kinds of decisions we make in our first years of life. One of these decisions has to do with living until we die or dying while we are physically living.

Since life is a gift to be enjoyed in its fulness, all that is needed if you, like the trick dog, have learned to "play dead," is to decide not to play dead any longer. Can it be that simple? Yes. You can give yourself permission to deserve the best life has to offer. You can begin to put into practice ideas suggested in this book that can help you live with joy all the days of your life. This living all your days means learning something new every day.

In recent years, vast research, numerous funded programs, and general public education have begun to turn the tide of how we see the living and learning potential of aging adults. Aging used to mean dependent, depressed, and often senile. Now we see that aging adults have vigorous capacities and desires to be independent, happy, and alert intellectually throughout their lives.

Continuing education courses in colleges and universities, opportunities to earn high school diplomas, Elderhostel's year-round programs, community adult education schools, all have widened horizons and challenged thinking. Many courses are offered, ranging in duration from a few hours to many weeks. Literally thousands of people enroll in courses offered by schools, colleges, universities and informal educational groups. Many churches also invite us to their adult classes and study groups.

In addition to courses open to adults, there are many other ways to learn: (1) Lessons in musical instruction (we know several people who have begun learning piano, violin, and guitar in their sixties/seventies; (2) library exploration in fields we know little of or in areas where we want to know more; and (3) clubs and associations for people of common interests—photography, hiking, bird watching, bridge, biking, and travel.

In preparing this book, we sent questionnaires to people asking for suggestions to help others age with a sense of joy. Almost all of them mentioned the importance of living and learning all of one's life. One said, "I make it a point to learn something new every day." This person is determined to see and hear what's happening around her and to learn all she can. Learning can be as informal as a bit of insight or knowledge added to one's life. It may be as relaxed as a few hours spent in an informal course on "The Life of the Arizona Indians" or "How to See the Stars." It may be a more rigorous series of classes to teach us French or Spanish. It may be a decision to write one's family history, to compose a piece of music, or to make needlepoint chair seats for a granddaughter's dining room. Learning can be as simple as discovering the name of a new flower, or as complex as writing a book, but the decision to live and learn all our life will bring a sparkle to our eyes and a warmth to our smile. It will make us much more interesting when our friends speak with us.

# Chapter 5

# Five Life Preservers

Have you ever felt as if you were drowning, not in water but in a sea of hopelessness? A drowning person needs a life preserver. This chapter describes five different kinds. Read about them, learn how to use them, and practice them each day: (1) Ask for what you want and need. (2) Enjoy what you have now. (3) Own your feelings. (4) Use the gift of time. (5) Every day give a gift away.

1) Ask for what you want and need. Don't expect people to guess. When we were infants and little children, it was our caretaker's job to know what we needed (food, clothing, cuddling, teaching). Before an infant learns verbal language, it has only its cries. Loving mothers soon learn to know the difference between cries for food, changing, pain, holding, etc. When children begin to talk and develop language skills, they are able to tell us many things they want and need. Caretakers must still anticipate some things needed by children since children do not have enough information or experience to know all their needs. Now if this process of meeting children's needs without indulgence or denial is unimpeded, then children grow up knowing what they need and knowing how to get their needs met through caring for themselves and being thoughtful of others.

All too often, however, this natural growing process is interfered with by older persons who, not having been properly cared for in their own childhood, are now sometimes unwilling and more often unable to take care of children who are their responsibility. Most parents do the best they can, giving to children the best of their own information and ways of parenting. But since parents were once children themselves and since their parents were often inadequate, these parents now are neglectful of their children. You may be a product of some misinformation about your own needs and how to meet them. The three untruths we have found most often passed on concerning needs are: (a) Don't ask for what you want or need. (b) Don't accept things if they are offered. (c) Don't refuse what is offered even if it is not what you need.

This first untruth carries with it the implication that it is selfish and self-centered to ask for what you want. It also carries with it a left-over childhood fantasy not appropriate to adult life: "Mommie will know." "Daddy will take care of me." They will guess. I don't have to ask. When we are grown and find that husbands, wives, close friends, sons, daughters, and nursing home attendants don't guess, we are hurt and often angry. We need to ask. This does not mean that each of us must demand our rights, see ourselves as the center of the world, and make unreasonable requests of those around us. It does mean that we each know more about ourselves than anyone else and that we each learn to ask others for what we want and need. "I'd like to come and see you." "May I have another pillow?" "I'd rather have lunch at 12, not 1." "I'd like more heat in my room." These are not egocentric demands. They are requests of people who have legitimate needs. Once we ask, we may have to do some follow-up, especially if we have asked a busy person. We may need to ask again. We also need to realize that our requests cannot always be granted. But they surely will never be granted if we don't ask. Most of the time we will be given what we want if we ask the right person at the right time in such a way that the response will be positive.

The second untruth is closely connected with the first. It usually goes on to imply, "People will think you're too eager, conceited, or grasping." In ancient China, the culture demanded that a polite person turn down the first offer of a gift or kindness. This turn-down had to be repeated and one was free to accept only if the offering was given a third time. Some of this same attitude was present in Victorian days and is still observed in parts of New England and the South. Whatever the reason for this quaint custom, it did take a great deal of energy on the part of those offering and on the part of the intended receiver. Rather than believing that this piece of folklore is a necessary courtesy, why not learn graciously to accept whatever is offered, if you really would enjoy it, rather than demurring with statements of unworthiness? It is a very simple thing to say, "Thank you," and accept the thoughtfulness of the giver.

If what is offered is not what you want or need, you may then get caught in believing a third untruth: "Don't turn anything down if it is offered." This untruth must account for the myriad unwanted gifts that lie unused in our houses, the bored countenances at numbers of luncheon or dinner parties, the listlessness that is evident when we see people together who are obviously mismatched and have nothing in common, and the half-hearted ways in which some people chair meetings or work on committees. These are all examples of people who wouldn't say no when they wanted to.

Whenever anyone offers us anything, they are in some way offering us a bit of themselves, a gift as it were, a gift of thought, time, courtesy. This offering should never be shunned. We should always thank them for their thought and courtesy. But we do not need to accept the concrete invitation, suggestion, or gift which they offer. The unwanted invitation may be graciously refused by, "How thoughtful of you to ask me. I won't be coming that day, but I know you and your guests will have a lovely time." The unwanted request to be a member or chair to a committee:

"How good of you to think of me. I'm going to say no because there are other things I want to do with my time, but
I want to wish you every success in finding another person." The unwanted gift—"Thank you for giving me____.
It's such a lovely color." (The gift can then be received with
graciousness, passed on to someone else who would appreciate it, or given to your favorite charity or church sale, the
giver not having been hurt by your so doing.) Simply give
yourself permission to turn down what you don't want or
need while at the same time being sensitive and courteous
to the giver.

2) Enjoy what you have now. To do this takes consciousness and discipline. It is easy to look forward when we are
young, and to look back to yesterday when we are older. It
is less easy to learn how to live *now*, grateful for yesterday,
looking forward eagerly to tomorrow, but living fully and
with gratitude today. Those who really live today will live
tomorrow more fully when tomorrow comes.

To enjoy what we have now means for some of us new
eyes, ears, and hearts. The great English mystic Evelyn Un-
derhill has a poem about looking and listening to life with
ears that hear and eyes that see:

I come in the little things
saith the Lord:
Not borne on morning wings
Of Majesty, but I have set My Feet
Amidst the delicate and bladed wheat
That springs triumphant in the furrowed sod.
There do I dwell, in weakness and in power;
Not broken or divided, saith our God!
In your strait garden plot I come to flower:
About your porch My Vine
Meek, fruitful, doth entwine;
Waits at the threshold, love's appointed hour.

I come in the little things
saith the Lord:
Yea! on the glancing wings
Of eager birds, the softly pattering feet
Of furred and gentle beasts, I come to meet
Your hard and wayward heart. In brown bright eyes
That peep from out the brake, I stand confest
On every nest,
Where feathery patience is content to brood
And leaves her pleasure for the high emprize
Of motherhood
There doth My Godhead rest.

I come in the little things
saith the Lord:
My starry wings
I do forsake,
Love's highway of humility take:
Meekly I fit My Stature to your need.
In beggar's part
About your gates I shall not cease to plead
As man to speak with man
Till by such art
I shall achieve My Immemorial Plan:
Pass the low lintel of the human heart.

If we begin to look anew at the little things of life, we
will see as children see—the commonplace as miracle. One
of the joys of being with children is their wonder, surprise,
and utter delight in rainbows, frogs, music boxes, stars,
hugs, and kisses. We, too, live in a world just like theirs, if
we will notice.

Yes, be grateful for yesterday, eager for tomorrow, but
live and enjoy today. When something is hard, painful, or
unpleasant today, we of course have to live through it, and
it is good to be in touch with and express our feelings

about the difficulties we encounter. But then, let's get on with the rest of the day rather than letting ourselves have a "bad day." Let us enjoy the hours that are not hard, painful, or unpleasant.

3) Own your feelings. In the first three chapters we spoke of the importance of feelings. We talked of life review, the healing of old memories, and the importance of finding a listening partner with whom we could share our feelings. In this chapter we simply point out that mental anguish and illness as well as physical disease and discomfort are sometimes caused by denying our true feelings and glossing over the depth of those feelings.

When we were children, our parents may have taught us that anger is not nice, sadness is unpleasant for others and fear is cowardly. To please our parents, then, we may have pushed away those feelings and buried our emotions in our unconscious. The truth is that parents are often uncomfortable with these so-called negative feelings and don't want to be around children who express them. What we should have been taught as children is that to be human is to experience the whole range of feelings. Then we should have been taught how to express the so-called negative feelings in ways that are appropriate. There are families where the so called positive feelings are rarely, if ever, expressed. These families are uncomfortable with hugs and kisses, with signs of joy and happiness, and expressions of love and affection. In such families, children soon learn to bury these positive feelings and later in life we perceive them as cold, unfeeling adults.

In almost every family one or more feeling is a "no, no." Most generally the "no's" are, "Don't be mad, sad, or scared." What the authors are suggesting as a third life preserver is that beginning now, you allow yourself to join the human race by owning all human feeling as part of yourself; that you accept the full range of feelings as part of your birthright. Once you have accepted your right to all feelings, you can then learn how to express them in ways that are appropriate to the situation, not harmful to others, and not harmful to you.

When you are feeling "mad," frustrated, irritated, upset, hurt:

a) Write a letter to the person with whom you are angry. Write this letter in child language and keep writing until your anger is dissipated. Read the letter over and over and then tear it up. Never send it. Writing will diffuse the energy built up by anger. Sending it will only be hurtful to the other person. After you have written the letter, you may then want to talk with the person about the issue, but because your rage will be gone, the other person will more likely be able to hear you. A letter can be written to a deceased person with whom we are still angry. It will have the same effect. We may then have an imaginary conversation to settle the issue in our own mind even though we can't actually talk with them.

b) Draw your anger on large pieces of newsprint. Use large crayons and draw until your anger has subsided. Keep the picture, date it, and look at it or draw another picture everytime you feel the "mad" coming on again.

c) Put an old pillow on your bed and imagine the person with whom you are angry on the pillow. Then take a hard stick or old tennis racquet and hit the pillow and keep hitting until you are calmed down. This exercise is more effective if you will make a noise as you hit. Yell or growl like an animal and then use words to tell the person on the pillow how "mad" you are. Before you start hitting, it is important to let your anger well up so you are in touch with real feelings and not just have a thought about anger. A good way to have feeling well up is to think about a specific instance when you were really angry with this person and then breathe deeply so you will not hyperventilate. Then let yourself feel more and more anger. Then do the hitting and noisemaking followed by strong words.

When you are feeling sad, depressed, blue, disappointed:

a) Cry as often and as long as you want to.

b) Write a story about a sad child and tell your story of sadness. (You are the little girl or boy.)

c) Put a doll, small pillow, or toy on your lap and let it represent your own inner child. Let this sad inner child tell you all about his or her sadness. Then, with the good mother or father within you, comfort the little child just as you would if you had an actual child there on your lap.

When you are feeling scared, timid, afraid, holding back:

a) Write a story as described above.

b) Use a pillow or doll as above.

c) Review your life to see when you first felt this same feeling of being scared. Then reconstruct that first scene, and this time instead of being scared, decide to bring a loving parent into the scene. With the protection of that parent beside you, change scare and fear into confidence and safety.

Since it is natural for children to express love and joy in both words and actions, we suggest that if you have been bottling up these expressions, simply allow yourself to do what comes naturally. You need first to find the untruth in your head and tell it to go away, that you no longer are going to give it power over you. Then live as you did when you were little, that is, spontaneously giving expressions of love and joy whenever you feel like it. Love and joy are contagious. Live them and let those around you catch their warmth.

4) Use the gift of time. We often hear people say, "I have time to kill." "I have more time than I need." "I don't know what to do all day." Our suggestion is to look at time as a gift that is ours to enjoy, use, and savor. There is an

old Pennsylvania Dutch expression, "The hurrier I go, the behinder I get." This describes much of the rushing world, and most of us have hurried too long. One of the joys of aging is that now we can take time—time for seeing anew, hearing as we have never heard before, savoring what we see and hear. We have time now to see God in the little things, to see people who need us and whom we need, to hear beautiful music, to taste food slowly, to savor our friends, our treasures, our mementos—time to live, and time to learn. Some of us are using time simply to wait for a Santa Claus or fairy godmother to bring the miracle package that will change our lives so that we may live happily ever after. Or we may be waiting for death to come and take us away from our cares and problems. The harsh truth is that there is no Santa Claus or fairy godmother with a miraculous package, bag, or wand. But. we can each be our own Santas and godmothers by opening ourselves up to the miracle of the joy of living all our days. Death will come to each of us in some tomorrow. There is no need to hurry it. Between now and then it is more fun to take time to enjoy.

5) Every day, give a gift away. One of the things people share is their love of gifts. From infancy to death most of us like to be given to, and sometimes there is added pleasure if we are surprised and do not know the gift is coming. We all like to know that someone has thought about us, and it is especially warming to have that thought come with a gift. Life would be more exciting if we all became gift givers. Most of us come in contact with people every day. Some of these contacts may be very casual (the mail carrier, grocer, delivery person, a passer-by on the street). Others may be more enduring (neighbors, table partner, bridge club players). Still others may be closer (friends, relatives, caretakers). But most of us do come in contact with people every day. What do we have to give? What do we

mean when we say, "Every day give a gift away"? Simply this: every one of us has the gift of ourselves; this is the most precious gift we can offer another person. When we offer ourselves to another, something happens that is like a tiny miracle. I offer you a little bit of myself when I smile at you as we pass on a street or in a store. If I know your name and I call you by name, you will likely have even more pleasure. If I touch your hand or arm with simplicity and friendliness, the warmth between us increases (unless you have been damaged early in life and believe that touching means cruelty or only a prelude to sexual encounter). Besides smiles, calling by name and touching, there are other gifts to be given. I may give you what has been called "a warm fuzzie," that is, something which you like to hear or have done. "You have beautiful eyes." "I like the dress or tie you are wearing." "Your smile is very warm." "I felt good when you backed my idea in the meeting this morning." "I'd like to have lunch with you." These are all positive ways of making others feel appreciated and good about themselves.

Suppose, however, that there are people we seldom see or don't see at all. Then our gift can be a telephone call, a card, a letter, a flower pressed into a note, a prayer on their behalf. Every day give a gift away. Try it. You'll like it.

# Chapter 6

# Talking to Yourself Is OK

Talking to ourselves is a phenomenon which has a powerful influence on the way we think, feel and behave. You may not be aware of it, but we all do it. The influence of this chattering which goes on inside our heads affects almost every area of our lives.

If you are aware of your interior dialogue and use it to your advantage—great! The following will help you become further aware of this powerful force. You can come to know what you say, how you say it, how you feel it, how you respond, and how it affects your behavior—and your life. You can find out what you need to do to make it more affirming and supportive.

This chapter will help you identify your messages, illustrate how these are likely to affect you, and outline eight steps to transform your internal dialogue into a most productive force in your life.

The way people talk to themselves is the single most significant thing that distinguishes winners—those who feel good about themselves and their lives—and losers—those who are dissatisfied, self-effacing, or critical about themselves. Become a winner!

1) Be aware of the way you talk to yourself.

    a) Listen to what you say. Begin by thinking for a moment what words flash through your head when you make a mistake. Some of the most common are:
- Stupid!
- What's wrong with you?
- Won't you ever learn?
- You're dumb.
- Can't you ever do anything right?

- What will people say?
- You're a disgrace.
- You should be ashamed of yourself.
- You're always messing up.
- You fool.
- You're no damned good.
- You're hopeless.

Next, listen to what you tell yourself when you have done something well. Common expressions include:

- Anyone could do that.
- You struck it lucky this time.
- There was nothing to it anyway.
- Don't be so pleased with yourself—
  pride goes before a fall.
- People won't like you if you're too smart.
- Now what are you going to do?

All of the expressions above are critical or down-grading, and encourage those who talk to themselves in these terms to feel inadequate or miserable. On the other hand, when winners make mistakes they are likely to say things like:

- You can fix it.
- Think what you need to do now.
- I can learn from this.
- What do I need to change?
- How can I correct it?
- It's OK to ask for help.
- You're good, you don't need to be perfect.

When they have done something well, winners affirm themselves with statements like these:

- Good for you.
- You did that well.
- I'm proud of you.
- You're a winner.
- I knew you could do it.
- You deserve to do well.

b) If you do not hear well, do this: Get yourself a small pad and pencil you can carry with you. Then, as you go about your daily activities, take a moment every now and again to listen to what you are saying in your head right now.

Whenever you get in touch with a message of any kind, write it down. For example, you are in a hurry and go to the shortest check-out line at the supermarket. All seems well until the person in front of you chats to the checker until she tells her the total of her bill. Only then does the woman begin to look for her checkbook, and then she takes the longest time to find a pen....Stop watching her; let yourself know what is in your head and write it on your pad.

As you get into the habit of being aware and listening, you will gradually get quite a list of messages. After a time, you can look over your list and see what themes emerge.

c) Become aware of the effect you have. As well as listening to the words you use, listen also to the effect and tone of your messages. When you make a mistake, do you talk to yourself in a loud, harsh tone, or is your voice like that of a caring and understanding friend? When you have done well, are your comments half-hearted, or are they enthusiastic and affirming?

As soon as you become aware of what you say and how you say it, you will be in a good position to decide whether you are treating yourself like a good friend or an undesirable enemy. You will also be able to identify how your conversation influences your feelings and behavior.

2) How your conversation influences you. Eric Berne, the developer of Transactional Analysis, identified these messages in our heads as "Parental tapes," which, like ra-

dio waves, are always present whether we consciously hear them or not. The way our parents talked to us when we were little children influenced the way we ourselves felt then. Our parental tapes determine how we feel about ourselves now. The way our parents related to us as children influenced our behavior then. The way we relate to ourselves now influences what we do now.

We can think of this in terms of the following diagram and illustrations, which show how easily we can get caught up in a vicious circle when the messages we give ourselves are judgmental or "mushy" rather than problem solving.

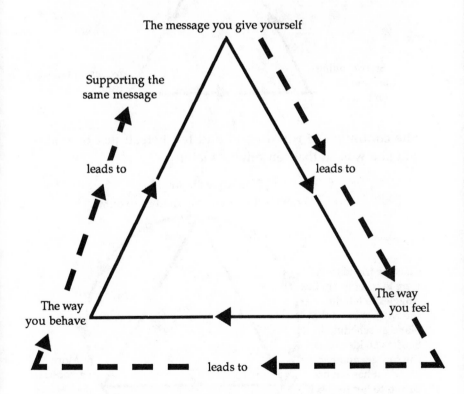

Let us imagine that three women—Sue, Jane, and Mary—were catching 8:00 AM planes from New York to Los

Angeles on the morning the clocks were advanced an hour for daylight saving time. They all had forgotten to advance their clocks. forward. Before leaving their houses, each one had realized her error. There was no possibility of getting to the airport on time. Their responses were as follows:

a) Sue's immediate response was:

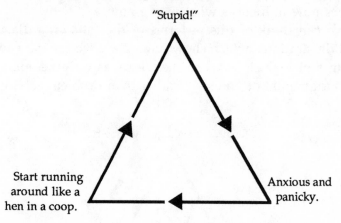

"Stupid!"

Start running around like a hen in a coop.

Anxious and panicky.

She continued to run around and tell herself just how stupid she was so that ten minutes later:

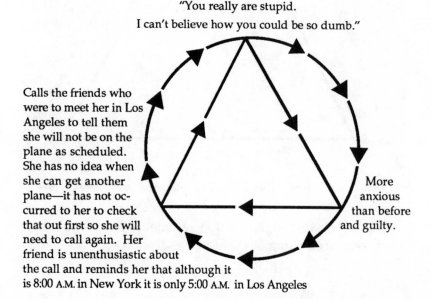

"You really are stupid.
I can't believe how you could be so dumb."

Calls the friends who were to meet her in Los Angeles to tell them she will not be on the plane as scheduled. She has no idea when she can get another plane—it has not occurred to her to check that out first so she will need to call again. Her friend is unenthusiastic about the call and reminds her that although it is 8:00 A.M. in New York it is only 5:00 A.M. in Los Angeles

More anxious than before and guilty.

b) Jane's immediate reaction was:

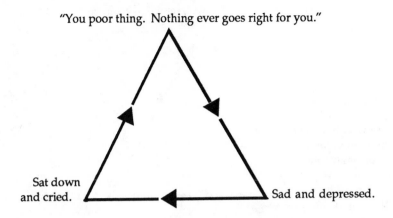

Ten minutes later she continued to pour out pitiful and helpless messages:

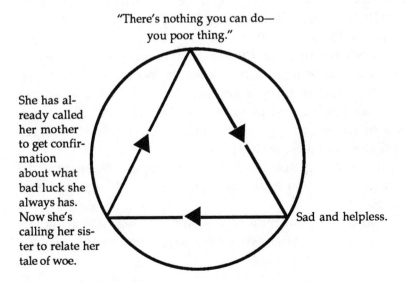

c) Mary's immediate response:

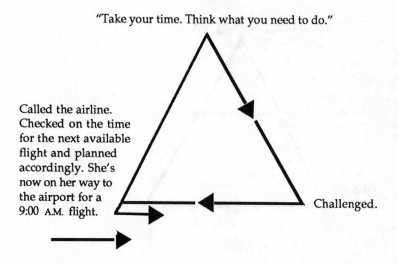

"Take your time. Think what you need to do."

Called the airline.
Checked on the time
for the next available
flight and planned
accordingly. She's
now on her way to
the airport for a
9:00 A.M. flight.

Challenged.

Sue's response, which is critical and nasty, and Jane's response, which is helpless and pitiful, both lead to feelings and behavior that are not problem solving and encourage self-destructive messages to be confirmed. A non-productive cycle keeps going. This saps energy and leads nowhere for some time.

Mary's response, on the other hand, accepts the reality of the situation without a put-down. It encourages her to use her resources to make a good decision so that she can get on with her life and use her energies constructively. Once she makes her new plans, the message in her head changes and she can go on with living.

3) Changing non-productive messages. When you do not like what you hear, the eight steps to change the messages are:

a) Identify the messages. Allow yourself to be aware of them no matter what they say. Some people benefit from making a list.

b) Evaluate them. Most probably some will be good

ones for you. This is fine—keep these. When you find any that are mean, nasty, or pitiful put downs, move to step three.

c) Think of good alternatives. Take the messages you want to change one at a time. Recall how you feel and what you do when you hear that message. Think of a good message for you under these circumstances. The illustrations of Sue, Jane, and Mary will serve as examples. Instead of telling herself how stupid she was as Sue did, or what a poor helpless person she was as Jane did, Mary told herself to think and plan so she could solve the problem and get on with life.

d) Decide how to turn off the old message. Although most of our old messages have been with us since childhood, and like radio waves are always with us, we can turn them off, refuse to listen, and refuse to believe them. Some people find the most effective turn-off procedure is to say "Stop it," "Go away," "I won't listen to you," etc. Others prefer a non-verbal, physical gesture such as stamping feet, sticking out tongues, or making faces; others prefer to make non-verbal noises such as a raspberry.

e) Practice changing stations. Imagine hearing the old tape, turn it off and plug in the new message. Examples:

- "You fool, you're always messing up."
- "I won't listen," said vehemently.
- "Think, you can get it right this time."

Then get two pieces of paper. On one write, "You fool, you are always messing up," and on the other write your good new messages. Examples:

- "You're a good thinker."
- "You can think."
- "You can do well."
- "You often get things right."

Now put the first piece of paper on the floor with the

messages facing up. Look at it, stand near it, and begin to despise it. Tell it it lies; you are not a fool; you don't always mess up, etc. Let it have it. If you feel like it, stamp on it or whatever else you feel like doing or saying. Finally, pick it up, rip it up, and literally dispose of it by burning it, flushing it, putting it in the outside garbage can.

f) Put this into effect daily. Whenever you are aware of any kind of nasty, helpless, or mean message, turn it off immediately and replace it with a positive, warm message.

g) Don't expect 100% immediate success. The old tapes have been in your head for many years and they are familiar. They will not change automatically. However, the sooner you recognize them and turn them off, and play a new recording instead, the more readily they will change. Any message you give yourself which is unsatisfactory can be changed by following these same steps.

h) Affirm yourself for each small change. When you start to find that you cut yourself down several times an hour and after a week or so you are doing it once or twice an hour, congratulate yourself on the change. For example, "You're doing great," "That's good, you've improved a lot," and "You're good, you don't need to be perfect." Keep up your practice and soon it will be only once or twice a day and then only occasionally.

The important thing is not whether we talk to ourselves in our heads—we all do; the important thing is how well we do it. The best messages we can give ourselves are appropriate to the situation. They affirm us as worthwhile thinking and feeling human beings. They encourage constructive living and problem solving.

# Chapter 7

# Your Body Speaks
# Its Mind

Not only do we communicate with ourselves through verbal messages in our heads, we communicate non-verbally within our bodies in several dramatic ways.

The most dramatic way is when our bodies figuratively shout with acute pain, "Look after me." The cry is so dramatic that people can scarcely fail to notice it. Next come those chronic or occasional aches which nag, nag, nag, until we pay attention. The mumblers and mild complainers are the little twinges, bloated and uptight feelings which precede the naggers and shouters, and often get ignored completely. Finally, there are the perfectly comfortable whispers that feel so good when we relax after stress, or are well after illness. Yet they are often taken for granted and unappreciated. Much of the time we simply ignore them and take them for granted.

The more we listen to the whispers and allow ourselves to be in touch and in tune with our bodies when they are comfortable, the more quickly we will become aware of the early signs they send warning us to tend, nurture, or restore ourselves before aches and pains appear. Prevention is far better than cure. However, we need to be knowledgeable about viable preventive measures and also be able to recognize problems as soon as they begin to emerge.

Check with yourself to see if you recognize the little signs of discomfort which almost always precede your aches and pains. When working with people with chronic headaches, for example, we ask, "What are the signs you get which precede the headache?"

Sometimes people know. More often, they do not. Some of the more common early signs include feeling more thirsty or hungrier than usual; feeling uncomfortable with a tender spot in the back of the neck; being overtired; craving certain foods; and being more sensitive to lights, noises and other petty annoyances.

When people are in touch with these signs, they can go back another and yet another step, until they get to the point where they can give their bodies what they need before they cry out for attention in some desperate and painful way.

Nancy, who had fairly frequent headaches, traced back her indicators and discovered that headaches always followed eating chocolate. Now she eats no chocolate and is more than happy not to do so in order to be quite free of headaches. Similarly, others have found that even small amounts of some hard liquors, red wines, vitamin E, coffee, sugar, strawberries, licorice, and other foods can trigger headaches which start about six hours after eating or drinking culprit foods or drinks.

Other people's chronic headaches have nothing to do with foods. Sometimes they are triggered by repressing anger, worrying over what someone might do, pushing too hard when rest was required and not taken, tensing certain eye or neck muscles, etc.

Only you can be observant. Look back to discover your early signals that a headache may be coming. Once you recognize the trigger foods or the early signals, you will be well on the way to preventing them, and to recognizing the importance of your body's energy—and its stoppage.

In tune with the rest of nature, our bodies are in perpetual motion. Even when we sleep, we tense and relax our nostrils and lungs each time we breathe, and our hearts with each beat. So long as we allow our organs to expand

and contract without holding back, our bodies function well, and without necessary pain. When we stop the flow, we hurt ourselves.

Think for a moment about your two hands. Look at them and notice exactly how they look, feel how they look, feel how they feel, and move your fingers around and notice how that feels. Now, clench your left fist. Hold it as tight as you possibly can for a timed minute. During the minute, remind yourself to keep it tight. At the same time, open and close your right hand at a steady pace.

At the end of the minute, gradually open and relax your left hand. Look at both hands, see exactly how they look and feel how they feel. Compare how your left hand looks and feels in comparison with your right. Almost certainly your right hand will look and feel the way it was before, while your left hand is likely to look stiff, whiter in some places, and redder in others. There will also be some mild discomfort for a few minutes.

The sages of yoga have identified irregular breathing as a major reason for physical distress. Whenever we are threatened in any way, our breathing pattern changes. We either hold onto most of the air in our lungs, thus only allowing small amounts of air to enter, or we exhale and inhale very quickly. In either case, we produce an imbalance of oxygen in our blood stream.

This imbalance causes stress which gathers in various places in our bodies. We all have our own preferred places. When this condition continues for extended periods, or at frequent intervals, it leads to pain and distress, and often to identifiable and serious tissue damage.

Sometimes this kind of stress leads to frequent problems such as aches in the head, neck, shoulders, or joints, which appear quite quickly. At other times, such as with those who get ulcers or heart attacks, extended periods of time may pass when symptoms can go unnoticed until a crisis occurs. By this time there is tissue damage.

The more familiar you become with how it feels to be at optimum comfort, and to recognize when the rumblings of mild symptoms begin, the more readily you will be in a position to allow your body to warn you when there is a small problem which needs to be noticed, attended to, and treated in a preventative way. Having recognized the results of energy flow and stoppages, you will be ready to see how your emotions and your energy are interrelated.

There is a relationship between our emotions and our energy. For example, whenever we are angry or scared, our bodies become flooded with adrenaline, which provides an immediate supply of energy. When we are happy, we have a good energy level, and when we are sad, our energy level is naturally low. When we find effective and appropriate ways to deal with the excess of energy accompanying anger or fright and the lack of energy which results from sadness, we can return to our natural energy level quite quickly.

Think for a moment about babies only a few months old. Everyone knows when they are angry—they yell and scream, pound their fists, kick their feet, go red in the face, and feel and look as if their blood is boiling. Then within a matter of minutes, the whole scene changes and they are quiet and peaceful, gooing and sleeping. Similarly, when they are scared they stiffen like a board and hold their breath until they are white in the face, and when they can hold onto their breath no longer. They let go and scream and expend their excess energy in much the same way as when they are angry.

When they are sad they have very little energy. They cry or whimper, often look pale, and hardly move at all except to curl up. It is as if they make themselves as small and still as possible. As with their angry and scared feelings, once they have expressed what they feel, they either become contented and comfortable again, or they go off to sleep.

As we grew from infancy to early childhood to adulthood, we needed to learn to channel our feelings in socially acceptable ways. We learned that we were not supposed to kick and scream whenever we were angry or scared, to curl up and cry whenever we were sad.

The tragedy is that many of us learned that we were not supposed to have any or all of those feelings. Somehow we were expected to be strong enough, brave enough, patient enough, and big enough to go on as if we felt just fine.

As a result of this training, many people feel guilty because they experience feelings. Others are afraid to express them. They hold on to them, swallow them, store them up, or repress them. They finally develop one of a multitude of physical problems or emotional problems such as depression, anxiety, bitterness, resentment, or guilt.

The most common psychological problems that emerge when feelings are stored up or repressed are depression and anxiety.

Often when people are angry, instead of doing something to use up their excess energy, they push it down and keep it inside. It does not go away. Instead, it requires more and more energy to keep it hidden. Gradually they become weary, think and move slowly, and talk quietly. They have problems with sleeping—either too long yet feeling tired all day, or sleeping too little. They have problems with eating too much or too often or hardly eating at all. Concurrently, they tend to have problems concentrating, withdrawing into themselves. They have repetitive thoughts about how depressed they are and how different it all would be if something had been different in the past.

Depression can be chronic or acute, mild or severe, connected with recent events or those of the past. It can come and go in a cyclical fashion, e.g., every Monday, each fall or Christmas, or it may be sporadic. Its victims can complain to everyone or they can hide it when they are with others.

They feel twice as bad when they are alone. Some people attempt to escape it by keeping busy or working all the time. Some resort to stimulants, alcohol, or drugs. Some wait it out or change their surroundings. Some find effective ways to deal with it.

The runner-up to depression on the emotional problems list is anxiety. As depression is connected with some unresolved feeling from the past, anxiety is connected with some feared outcome in the future. Just as depression is linked to the "If only I hadn't, they hadn't...If only it had been different," etc., so anxiety concerns itself with "What if...some terrible tragedy occurs." Depression generally starts with repressed anger. Anxiety is almost always connected with fear.

In an airplane coming down for a crash landing, your natural reaction would be fear, and your body would react in tune with that fear. You would almost certainly stiffen up, grab hold of the armrest, automatically flooding the body with adrenaline, and shake with fear. If by chance you survived the landing, you would either sit or shake, or be up and out of that plane in double quick-time.

When you only *fear* that a plane is going to crash, your body reacts in exactly the same way. Sometimes people experience anxiety far in advance of the event, either in their waking hours or in their dreams.

The characteristics are similar with any form of anxiety. Physical reactions are identical, whether fear results from a reality scare or anxiety develops from an anticipated or imagined dreaded consequence.

Feared outcomes may be connected with physical danger, loss of any kind, anticipated consequences or criticisms. When this continues, eating and sleeping habits are affected, concentration abilities decrease, and thoughts are often muddled. We become preoccupied and sometimes obsessed with our fear; we may hyperventilate, shake, develop rashes or bad breath, talk constantly or hardly at all, start sentences and not finish them, have frequent nightmares, or develop phobias.

As with depression, anxiety can be chronic or acute, vary from relatively mild to very serious, be cyclical or sporadic.

Often by using one or more of the methods outlined in the next chapter, the problems of depression and anxiety can be dealt with. At other times when they are severe, it is advisable to get professional help. More information on when to seek help and how to find a competent therapist will be found in Chapter 14, "When You Need Help."

# Chapter 8

# Taking Care of Yourself

Are you your own best friend? Do you know how to love yourself? If so, you are already taking good care of yourself. This chapter will support many of the things you are doing.

If, however, you have not been taking care of yourself as well as you could, this chapter will help you do better. The more you do it, the more you will like it. The better you take care of yourself the more you will appreciate the other people in your life.

When we were born we had a caretaker, usually our mother, whose job it was to care for our physical and emotional needs. Our only way to ask for help was to cry; our mothers quickly learned what our cries meant—the need for changing, holding, feeding, etc.

Gradually we learned words, and then how to put those words together to ask for what we wanted and needed. If we had good parenting and our needs were met in a loving way, we were then able to care more and more for ourselves, until finally we could leave our parents' home and make a home for ourselves and our own children.

In some people, however, the transition from total dependence to complete independence is interfered with by various outer and inner disruptions. Such people never learn to care for themselves as much as they need to, and they may forever be looking for some "good mommy" who will appear miraculously and take care of them for the rest of their lives. Some people in their seventies, eighties, or nineties who are perfectly able to care for themselves do not do this because they want a fairy godmother to bring them what they need.

In theory, miracle mothers could appear but in fact this is not likely! The reality is that whatever our early parenting deficiencies, we all need to learn to take good care of ourselves right now. We need to be our own best friend. Here are five ways to do that:

1) Eat for health. Many people eat to eat, eat to have something to do, eat because it's mealtime, eat because they are bored, or eat without being aware that they are eating. Eating for health is different. Food is for our bodies' nourishment, growth and strength. If we eat "funny" foods, junk foods and non-foods, if we fill our stomachs with salt, sugar, caffeine, additives, preservatives, and fats, we can expect to have aches and pains and a dwindling supply of energy. If, on the other hand, we eat well-balanced meals along with an adequate supplement of vitamins, minerals, and amino acids, we can more likely expect healthy tissues, strong muscles, and feelings of well-being. It is unfortunate that many physicians have little knowledge of nutrition. It is also unfortunate that many food faddists frighten us into unbalanced, dangerously lopsided diets. But sound nutritional information is neverthe- less available.

We like *Nutrition Almanac* from Nutrition Search, Inc. and authored by John D. Kirschman and Lavon J. Dunne. It is a McGraw-Hill paperback and sells for $10.95. It covers, Nutrition and Health; Sources of Calories; Nutrients and How they Function Together; Food Composition Chart; Ailments, Stressful Conditions and Nutrition and a final section on Herbs.

2) Move your body. Twenty minutes of continuous exercise in such things as walking, swimming, running, or biking is considered to be ideal for most adults if such exercise is done three to five times a week. Nothing contributes to pain, stiffness, and atrophy as much as disuse. So the rule is "Keep moving as much and as long as you can." Even if

you are at an irreversible point and even if you are in a wheelchair, you can still do some isometric exercises with your hands, feet, or head.

3) Rest. Most people will agree that a good night's sleep is part of a sensible lifestyle. The number of hours people sleep is widely variable. Some get along quite well on a few hours of sleep; others need eight hours or more. Sleep researchers have found that the quality of sleep is as essential as the amount of sleep, and most people seem to find what is best for them.

It is equally true, however, that for untold numbers of people sleep has its problems: inability to fall asleep, wakefulness during the night, awakening too early in the morning, inability to awaken on time, restlessness during sleep and fatigue when waking in the morning. Innumerable pills to help us sleep and sleep better are advertised and consumed. Better yet, plenty of good advice can be found. Here are our ideas:

•Don't take medication except, in a crisis, for temporary relief. Sleeping pills are usually habit-forming and generally lose their effectiveness rather quickly.

•Don't get upset because you have sleep problem. Solve the problem instead.

Common causes of sleep problems are:

•temperature in the room—too hot or cool;

•moisture—too dry or too damp;

•food—too stimulating (caffeine, sugar, alcohol); overly rich fat; too little or too much; insufficient nutritions; emotional stress—worry, tension, fear, loneliness, depression, anxiety, over-tiredness.

Sleeping at night is accepted as a good idea by almost everyone, but we have found frequent resistance to our suggestion that people have a midday rest. Nevertheless, a midday rest is a wonderful way to break up the day's activities and allow our bodies to wind down before continuing the afternoon and evening program. It is not self-indulgent or lazy to have a midday rest. It is a way of being refreshed, of preventing over-tiredness, and of gaining renewed energy for the rest of the day.

4) Have fun. According to one psychological study, we all have three internal ego structures (Parent, Adult, and Child). Our Parent function tells us what's right and wrong—the do's and don'ts which take care of us and other people. The Adult function stores information and makes it available to us when we need it, rather like a computer data bank and processor. The Child function is our feelings, and among other things is the fun-loving part of us, the simple, accepting, trusting, free part. When we are growing up, this part of our child is sometimes squashed by older people who are intent on making us into responsible, obedient, hardworking, good adults. Somewhere along the way, the happy, free, fun-loving child gets lost. We become responsible, obedient, hardworking and good grown-ups, and we may also become overserious, guilty, depressed, and unhappy. Taking good care of yourself includes recovering your lost child and learning again how to have fun. It is never too late to start to find your lost child. Here's how:

a) Make a fun list. List everything you have ever wanted to do. Don't think about it. Just list it.

b) Give yourself permission from your caring parent to do anything on that list that is not going to hurt you or anyone else. Try as many things as you want to and keep doing them until you see what is really fun for you now.

c) Add to your list as you think of other possibilities or see other people doing things you would like to try. If in your head you hear comments like "Don't be childish." "You're acting silly." "What will people think?"—tell that voice to stop talking and replace it with another voice that says, "I like to see you have fun." "You deserve to play." "It's great to see you so happy."

d) Find other people to play with you. They have been waiting for you to ask them to have fun with you. Here are some ideas from fun lists we have seen:

- Buy an ice cream cone.
- Wear socks that don't match.
- Go barefoot through the grass or sand.
- Learn to bike, swim, play tennis, sail, play bridge, or a musical instrument.
- Join a group to do clay modeling, ceramics, or other art forms.
- Sit in a shopping mall and make silly remarks to yourself about people who look funny to you.
- Make faces at yourself in your bedroom mirror.
- Soak in a hot bathtub with only candlelight in the room and music playing in the background.
- Try new hairstyles.

5) Checkups. In his book *Your Body Speaks Its Mind*, Dr. Alexander Lowen says our bodies tell us, through our fatigue, discomfort, and pain, when they need to be looked after. If we are willing to take good care of ourselves, we can often prevent bodily distress. Some physicians suggest that we care for ourselves by having a yearly or every other year physical checkup after we reach the age of forty. Such checkups can often forestall serious illness because they make it possible to solve simple problems in early stages. If there is a physical problem, we need to know of it as soon as possible and take care of it.

Eating for health, moving, resting, relaxing, and having fun will prevent many physical problems; regular physical checkups will often prevent more serious illnesses.

Chapter 9

# When You Are in Physical Pain

What do you want when you are in pain? Relief, of course, but relief comes more readily when you believe in what is suggested—medication, prayer, herbal potions, surgery. Strong belief—potent relief.

The authors have taught many clients how to reduce physical pain through relaxation and imaging. We discuss four methods that you, too, can use. But first a few words about diagnosis and medication.

Pain is real, it is distressing, and it needs attention. In one sense pain is a good friend. It watches out for us, letting us know when something is wrong and needs our attention. When your body gives you a signal, be good to yourself and get problems checked out medically. Whenever possible, establish the cause—only then will you and your advisers be able to make the best judgment about treatment.

1) Medication. The first thing many people want to do is to take something to relieve the pain. We have only to watch American television for one day to discover how our culture is preoccupied with pill-taking. Sometimes it is wise to take pain reducing drugs and sometimes not.

In the previous chapter we included a segment on the importance of periodic and preventive checkups and of choosing a physician who is willing to discuss your condition with you. If possible find one who has a holistic approach to medicine. Whenever your physician prescribes drugs, ask about the possible side effects. Establish also what the medication is designed to do, e.g., whether to help cure the cause, prevent the spread of infection, hasten healing, or reduce pain. You have a right to know. Also, ask about the addictive potential before you take any medication. If you have any uneasiness about this at all, discuss it with your physician and ask if there are other alternatives. While many prescriptions or over the counter drugs are frequently helpful and sometimes essential for our well being, they are not always the best. There are other forms of treatment. The first of these is relaxation.

2) Relaxation. Recent research has discovered that beta endorphins manufactured in the brain are powerful natural pain killers—more powerful than morphine. The key is to know how to release these to do their work.

Although much is still unknown about the effective use of endorphins, we do know that deep relaxation, hypnosis, and laughter are effective releasing agents.

One of the most effective ways of becoming relaxed is to find a comfortable place and give your total attention to your breathing. Notice if it is fast or slow, deep or shallow, even or uneven. There is no need to change your breathing at this point. Simply notice how fast, how deep, and how even it is. Notice how far toward your abdomen you feel movement as you exhale and as you inhale; notice the movement of your clothes on your body; notice how far toward your shoulders you are aware of movement as you breathe. Take all the time you need to become aware of these movements.

Notice how the air feels in your nostrils as you inhale and exhale. Notice how it is different as you draw air into your body and as you send it away. Be aware of the movements of all the thin hairs in your nose; listen to the sound of the air as you exhale and as you inhale. Notice now if there is any difference in your breathing. It may be slower or shallower; it may be more or less even. The more relaxed you become the less oxygen you need.

Concentrate now on inhaling comfort and exhaling stress or tension. With each inhalation feel your body becoming more and more at peace, more and more relaxed, more and more comfortable. Allow every exhalation to take you to a deeper and deeper level of relaxation.

Another method which is widely used and which some people prefer is to start either at your toes or at the top of your head and concentrate on relaxing one part of your body at a time.

If you start with your toes, move up to concentrate on your feet, ankles, legs, knees, etc., until you reach the top of your head. If you start with your head simply reverse the order.

A third common way is to make yourself comfortable, close your eyes, and imagine you are in a wonderful relaxing place—at the beach, in a hammock, in the mountains, or by a waterfall. Concentrate on being there. Smell the place, look at it, touch it, taste it, hear the sounds that are there and become at one with that place.

We suggest you experiment with these methods and find which one you prefer. You may choose to use a combination of two or all three or add anything else you know about relaxing. Relaxation is even more effective for pain relief when it is combined with imaging.

3) Imagination and Visualization. We outline four methods of visualization and imagination that may be used for pain reduction or healing. They move from simple to advanced.

The first, and simplest (a), may be used at any time and in any place without any previous preparation. It is effective for pain reduction and is especially recommended for chronic aches and pains. It may be used for just a few minutes or for as long as the occasion warrants.

The second method (b) is more specific and yet quite simple. It is particularly helpful when your pain is in a part of your body which has a partner, as it were, on the other side of your body and which is not affected with pain, e.g., when your right elbow hurts and your left is fine. This requires a little imagination.

The third (c) is more detailed and specific. It takes varying amounts of time depending upon the severity and stubbornness of the pain and the ease with which you allow your imagination and visualization to work for you. It is often effective for severe headaches, minor arthritic conditions, and the like.

The fourth (d) can be as complicated as you want to make it. It does involve careful thought and planning and generally needs to be used regularly over a period of time. This is a method to use as an adjunct to medical procedures and where there is already tissue damage.

Method a. Find the most quiet and most comfortable place you can. If this is in a bus or behind a busy desk, that is all right. Take a few moments to get in touch with your breathing and relax, using any method that works for you. As you do this, imagine you are inhaling healing and energy and exhaling tension. If, after a few moments, you have difficulty relaxing any part of your body, tighten it and then let go. Doing this two or three times often hastens your relaxation.

Now take a moment or two to see the most beautiful, gentle, and healing color you can imagine. It does not matter what color it is or if it changes or remains the same—simply let yourself know what it is. (If you do not visualize colors, allow yourself to remember the color you want and think about that color.)

Next, imagine yourself surrounded by this beautiful color; draw it all around yourself as if you were in a big cocoon. If you like, you can fill the whole room or area where you are with it. having done that, start to inhale it. Watch or imagine this color with all its healing qualities come into your body through your nostrils to your lungs;

from your lungs take it with the oxygen into your heart and bloodstream, and send it throughout your body, from the top of your head to the tips of your toes.

As you do this, allow the color to bring comfort, tenderness, and the healing it symbolizes for you. This will reduce your pain and renew your energy. Continue to have the color surround and fill your whole body, yet focus on its working where you have the pain.

If you like, give the pain another color—one which symbolizes pain, discomfort, and tension to you. With each exhalation watch that color leaving your body. Watch it moving far away from you and disappearing in the distance. Replace the painful color with the one filled with comfort. Continue to do this so long as you need; then stretch your body as you gradually open your eyes and look around the room.

Method b. Find the most comfortable place you can. Sit or lie down and relax, using any method you choose. If surrounding yourself with a symbolic color appeals to you, do that. If not, simply become as relaxed as you can.

Take a moment or two to focus upon and become more aware of your pain. Look at it from the outside and then from the inside and see what it looks like. See or imagine the colors, the movements, the bones, tissues, joints, veins, or whatever. When you have done that and have a clear image, move to the corresponding place on the other side of your body and see how that looks from all aspects.

Having done that, be aware of how they look different, e.g., the hurting side may look red and jumpy while the other side may look a pale rose color and have only very slow movements. Or, one side may be full of knots made with rusty looking wire and the other may have threads intertwined.

Now go back and focus on the painful side. Watch it and gradually have it change in appearance so that it slowly comes to look more and more like the healthy side. The process generally takes between five and ten minutes. It does not matter how the change takes place—simply watch it happening.

When we (the authors) have used this method with ourselves and clients, sometimes the color is the first thing to change and sometimes the last. The sequence is irrelevant. The process of watching and feeling the change take place is the significant part of this healing method.

Method c. Once again begin by taking time to be as comfortable and quiet as possible. Allow yourself to relax using any method you want and then focus on your pain. Let yourself know how long it is, how wide, how deep; what shape it is; what color and the kind of texture it has. Take all the time you need to be aware of the details.

Elaine experienced her pain as being three inches long, a half-inch wide, and two inches deep. It had the shape of a block with extremely sharp edges. It was black with some dark green veins in it similar to those in marble; its texture was hard, like a rock. In some places it was almost shiny and smooth, and yet it was more like sandpaper in others. It was very heavy and felt as if it were filled with mercury.

Robert experienced and saw his pain in several parts, each one being a long, thin, arrowlike rod about ten inches long and an eighth of an inch wide and deep, with needle-like points that were red and flashed like lightening. The texture was smooth, and the rods looked like spokes from a bicycle wheel.

Simply allow yourself to describe how you experience your pain and how it looks and feels to you. Your description may be quite literal, like the first description by Elaine, or it can be symbolic, as it was with Rosemary, who described her tooth ache as being six feet long.

Once you have your image and description clearly in mind, concentrate on watching it decrease in size. Watch carefully until it is half its original size, then one quarter in size, then one eighth in size. Notice too how it changes shape. It may become a smaller version of the original or it may reduce by changing its general shape. Notice any changes of shape, color, or texture as it becomes so tiny that you can scarcely see it.

At this point decide how you will have it leave your body. This can be through any of your body openings or through the pores of your skin. Watch it leave and continue to watch it until it disappears. Check to see how you feel. What has happened to the pain?

In our experience in working with a number of clients with headaches and other chronic aches and pains, about seventy-five percent have said their headaches had gone by the time the tiny particle disappeared. All but four of the others reported feeling much better.

Sometimes, after pain is diminished or alleviated by this method, it returns after a time. When this happens it is almost always in a milder form. With a very stubborn pain, e.g., arthritic shoulder pain or bursitis, you may need to repeat the process a few times until the pain is cured.

This method often works better when someone else guides the person with the pain by asking the questions and eliciting responses from the sufferer. If you have headaches or other nagging pains, we suggest you have a friend sit down with you to guide you so that you can concentrate on doing the procedure while not needing to think of all the steps.

Method d. This method, which is often useful as an adjunct to medical treatment, requires thought and planning before being put into effect. One of the authors has used this with several clients whose problems fall into one of three categories:

• a problem for which there is no known cure, e.g., venereal herpes;

- medically diagnosed problems that may require surgery if they do not improve with a change in diet or drugs, e.g., ulcers;
- various stages of cancer.

Our bodies have self-healing capacities that we know very little about at a conscious level. We do know, however, that we can encourage self-healing to take place by utilizing the healthy parts of our bodies.

Following are steps to take in preparation for Method d, with illustrations and examples of symbols used by participants who have benefited from this method:

a) Think about the nature of the problem and the form it takes then think of a symbol to represent the problems. Examples:

- herpes—a series of tiny volcanos ready to erupt at any time;
- an ulcer—an underground dump site which smolders constantly; and
- abdominal cancer—a parasitic plant ready to flourish by sapping nourishment from anything it can find. Make the symbol your own.

b) Decide upon which healthy system, such as your respiratory system, digestive or circulatory system, or which healthy part of your body you will use to form an army to prepare to attack and overcome the problem.

c) Plan how the system you choose can become an army which is powerful enough to win the battle for health against the enemy. For example, for herpes you could choose the circulatory system. In the battle against herpes each red blood cell is to be a miniature squirt gun which contains a powerful potion for disintegrating and demolishing volcanos. Each white blood cell which follows is a salve which not only picks up debris from fragmented volcanos, but also promotes healing and feels good.

d) Decide how you will eradicate every piece of the problem from your body, e.g., through your urine or your exhalations.

To be successful with this method, you must ensure that your army has sufficient power and adequate weapons to deal with the symbol you choose for the problem. It would be useless to have the problem seen as a great forest fire and the respiratory system provide an army of a gentle breeze to attempt to turn the fire back on its tracks.

Once you have decided upon your symbols and method of attack, find a comfortable place, relax using any method you want, and visualize or imagine your problem in its symbolic form. Muster your army and put it to work. Allow the army all the time it needs to complete its task. Then concentrate on how you will ensure that you eliminate every trace of the problem.

Do this exercise daily for a minimum of three weeks. As improvement takes place, change the size or nature of your symbol accordingly. With problems like herpes and ulcers, the expectation is that they will go into remission. If, at a later time, there are any warning signs that the problem may be recurring, immediately reactivate your program.

With cancer, continue to use the program daily until your checkups show you have no further signs. If the cancer is one that tends to go into remission with the expectation of future problems, continue your program until remission takes place, and then develop a new program to keep it there.

# Chapter 10

# When You Have a Loss

When we lose something or someone we love, part of us dies. Our whole being experiences shock and we grieve for our loss. That grief must be handled gently, lived with, and worked through effectively.

Dealing with grief effectively is the process by which we come to accept the reality of the loss, live through and deal with the feelings we have in relation to it, and reach the point where we can lay grief to rest in such a way that we are free to get on with and live the rest of their lives.

Some people, the fortunate ones, are willing and able to do whatever they need to do so that the loss, serious as it may be, does not ruin the meaning of all they still have. Even so, it takes about a year for the major part of the grief work to be done.

A second group of people seems to grieve for years. Generally, this occurs when, for any number of reasons, they do not put their loss to rest. Instead, they allow themselves to be preoccupied or haunted. They feel miserable and go on suffering about what they do not have. They do not accept or use the opportunities and the resources they have.

A third group of people appears to have very little reaction to losses. They go about their business as if everything is just fine, when actually they have ignored and repressed their feelings.

Universal grief reactions to important losses are shock and disbelief, followed by sadness, anger, and fear, although not necessarily in that order. In addition, there is almost always a sense of guilt, often depression or anxiety, and sometimes physical illness.

Whether a loss or tragedy is sudden or expected, a shock reaction does occur. Often when people know the inevitable, there is still a period before they accept the reality. "Oh, no!" is probably the most common response when people hear bad news.

The reactions of family members, colleagues, school children, and many others to the explosion of the shuttle Challenger in 1986 illustrate this. The overall reaction was a hushed silence. There was virtually no movement; many people looked as if they were gasping for air as they stared for a few moments before they clasped each other. Only later did they begin to cry.

Once the reality of loss is accepted, the grieving process can begin. This process is work. It is never easy, nor is it pleasant in any sense of the word. Those who pass through it most easily and effectively are those who are willing to allow themselves to feel what they feel, express those feelings and let them go.

These people are most likely to cry when they are sad. They accept the fact that they are angry. They either talk about their anger or thrash it out. They may yell, scream, and write about it, or they may become involved with energetic physical activities. When they feel afraid of their situation, they will get the information and reassurance they need from friends or professionals. If they feel guilty, they will evaluate that, examine themselves and if necessary make amends; they will be willing to seek forgiveness from God or others and forgive themselves if need be.

From time to time, and especially at the beginning stages of the process, there are likely to be periods when they do not know how they are going to feel from one moment to the next. There will be mornings when they wake up feeling better than they have in a long time. Then, suddenly without any apparent cause, they may feel awful. At other times they may begin the day feeling terrible, then feel just fine.

This period of ambivalance and unpredictable feelings may be the most difficult of all. However, those who learn to live with themselves throughout their ups and downs do realize that these too will pass.

Some people have excessive problems with grieving; they may feel overwhelmed, helpless, or hopeless for long periods of time. Some, by repressing their feelings, appear to be indifferent. It is almost certain that these people either have difficulty in dealing with their feelings, enabling the emotions to leave so that other feelings may take their place, or they scare themselves in some way.

In Chapter 7 we described effective ways of dealing with feelings and how to let them go. In Chapter 6 we explained how to identify unhelpful messages and the steps to take to replace these messages with constructive and caring ones. Since problems with grieving are so common, re-reading those chapters may be helpful

Some examples of the ways people  hinder themselves in dealing with their feelings, and the alternatives they have, are as follows:

Long after the loss of an arm a woman feels depressed and tearful as she dresses. She says to herself, "I wonder why I'm so upset today." Suddenly she remembers, "Oh, of course, it is Tuesday. I always feel terrible on Tuesdays because that was the day I had my accident"; this gives her an excuse to keep on feeling bad all day and every Tuesday for the rest of her life.

On the other hand, she may decide enough is enough. Instead of looking for a rationalization for feeling depressed whenever she thinks about the loss of her arm, she can say to herself, "Enough of that." She can give herself a moment to think about something she has that she feels good about, something she can appreciate, enjoy, or laugh about.

Every time she remembers the pain of the loss, she

should remind herself that the loss itself was painful enough. She has no need to punish herself by dwelling on it any more. Today is the time to live with all the other limbs, organs, and resources she has.

A widow who tells herself over and over again, "Life is meaningless without a man," or "You'll never make it alone" is likely to feel afraid and anxious. She is likely to act in an inadequate way, only proving time and time again that she *will* never make it or that life *is* meaningless. She may become frantic in her search to find a man and run the risk of grabbing any man she can get, no matter how unsuitable .

Alternative positive messages like, "You can make it," "You're a fine person in your own right," "You're worth taking care of," are likely to make a great difference in the way she feels and in her adjustment to a new way of life.

A man who has been forced to retire against his will can make the remainder of his life miserable if he constantly tells himself, "I'm no good unless I'm working," "I always knew I would get the axe one day," "There must be something wrong with me." So long as he continues these messages he is likely to feel inadequate, depressed, and worthless, and unlikely to find anything to change his situation. Messages like, "You can do new things," "You have lots of choices now," "You are free to get another job," "You have a lot to give," "People will be glad to discover you," said often and sincerely, will result in a change in his feelings, energy level, attitudes, and opportunities.

Whether losses involve physical illness or accident, status, independence, home, other people, or love, the grieving process is essentially the same. When you have losses—be good to yourself. Allow yourself to grieve. Tell yourself time will heal.

When people have serious losses or several losses in quick succession, it is to their advantage to seek skilled professional help. We have written more about this in Chapter 14. In our opinion the wisest policy when having problems in grieving is to seek a skilled therapist who does short-term crisis intervention without the use of drugs. A few sessions with a good therapist may save months and even years of suffering.

# Chapter 11

# So Alone, So Lonely

Loneliness is not reserved for the aging, although aging often increases the pain of loneliness. In our younger days we often ran away on a buying trip, or escaped through the movies, a vacation, a club meeting, or a "keep busy" activity. When we returned home, we were often out of energy and too tired to cope with our loneliness. Now that we are older, we may have less money and even less energy to run. We feel our loneliness even more.

Loneliness seems to be an almost universal problem. It is felt by infants, growing children, young persons, adults in the prime of life, and finally the elderly. No circumstance of life mitigates it. Money, education, beauty, power, talent, uprightness of character—nothing protects us from the experience of loneliness. But there is much about loneliness which if understood will alleviate its pain and bring healing to the wound it inflicts.

As we begin to understand ourselves, it is important to separate the concept of loneliness from that of aloneness. To be alone is to be by oneself. This may be a matter of choice, and even if we do not choose to be alone, being alone does not necessarily mean being lonely. Aloneness is a physical matter. It is being in a physical location by oneself. Loneliness, on the other hand, is a feeling which may be experienced either when we are by ourselves or when we are with other people. It carries with it a sense of separateness, isolation, and abandonment, and is often accompanied by feelings of inferiority and rejection—"Something is wrong with me." Aloneness can be a time for rest, relaxation, creativity, fun, or disciplined work. When we are alone, we can refresh our bodies with a warm bath or stretch out on a sunlit beach. We can take off our shoes and walk barefoot through the morning grass or feel the autumn leaves fall on both sides of our feet. We can write poetry, memoirs, letters to friends, or stories. We can practice a musical instrument, bake cookies, write reports, refinish furniture, watch the return of Canada geese, listen to music, or sit and simply be. When we are alone, we can take time to see, hear, smell, and touch the miraculous world in which we live. We can appreciate it, give thanks for it and celebrate the joy of living. We can be more aware of ourselves and everything else than if we were with another person chattering on as we are so wont to do. To be alone is to have endless opportunities for new dimensions in life and its living.

To be lonely, on the other hand, is to be plugged into self-pity, to feel oneself boxed into a place that seems to have no exit: the small, small world of one's own ego, the miniscule place of rejection and isolation. Here we believe ourselves to be helpless, loveless, and hopeless. Whatever is outside our dark world, whatever exists of beauty, love and warmth, seems non-existent. We may know in our heads that sunsets, flowers, bird song, green valleys, music, painting, children's faces, and heroic spirits are all beautiful, but we feel no beauty. We may know that love is in the world, but we feel no love. We may know that life has some meaning, but we feel meaningless and desolate. We feel insulated from all other men and women, from all other reality. If some well-meaning person tries to enter our isolation and tell us what is outside our prison, we know this person does not really understand, and we sink even further into our abyss of darkness and despair. To be truly lonely must surely be one of earth's blackest hells.

Perhaps most people experience this depth of loneliness only occasionally. But for those who do struggle with its depression and isolation, five steps may be helpful.

1) "This too will pass." Many people who suffer physical or emotional pain believe it will last forever. It is this "always" and "forever" that defeat us. We are consumed by the belief that we are helpless to change our condition and that for the rest of our days we will experience the depth and agony of the pain we are now enduring. With our intellect we may know that it is otherwise, but we allow ourselves to be swallowed up by the dark waters of despair. Only a stronger and more positive way of thinking will conquer negative thoughts like these. When we feel the desolation returning, we must say over and over, "I feel this now. It is not going to last forever. It will go away. This too will pass."

2) "You are lovable." The thought patterns just discussed are usually those of rather outgoing personalities. Introverted people have a different way of experiencing loneliness. Here is a likely pattern of false messages that keep going on in their heads.

a) Don't tell people how you feel.

b) Act strong, as if you don't need anyone.

c) Try hard to please everyone else, but no matter how hard you try, you'll never be able to do it.

d) There must be something wrong with me, or people would want to be with me.

e) It's so easy for others to make friends. Life isn't fair to me.

f) If I knew what was wrong with me, I'd change it.

People who believe in these untruths always put a lot of energy into them: "I just knew my life would be like this." "It always has been lonely." They put little energy into working on change. For them, change will come only when they refuse to poison themselves by believing these six untruths.

3) Take charge of your depression. Whether a person is extraverted or introverted, this step is essential. You have

already begun to do this when you admit that the time will come when you will not feel lonely as a way of life. This admission will allow you to take further charge, by facing the pain of the loneliness you now feel rather than trying to escape that pain.

4) Face your feelings straight on. Feel the pain, know that even though it will pass, now you are willing to look at it with its ramifications to see what is so awful and what is so devastating. This may sound redundant, but it takes real "stick-to-itiveness" to face one's inner self with such questions as: When did I first feel lonely in my life? Who was with me or who was not there with me? Whom did I want to be with me? How is this moment of loneliness like those early times of loneliness? Have I in some un-conscious way "set it up" to be lonely now? Are there those I could be with now if I chose to be? What awful thing do I expect to happen if I am lonely? These and other questions are a way of probing one's inner self and coming to new self-realization. The answer to any one of them could be the beginning of an imaginative story. By writing this story we will learn much more about ourselves. Any of our written answers, or our story writing can lead us to other insights which can ease our pain if they are accepted as a real part of our own life story.

5) Make the changes necessary to move out of isolation. You have already begun to do this by following steps 1–4, just above. Now you may choose further steps:

a) Let go of your fantasy about finding a surrogate and all-loving parent (usually mother) who will make up for what you didn't get from your own mother or father.

b) Give up believing in Prince Charming or the beauti-ful Princess who will give you eternal happiness if only you are with him or her forever.

c) Stop telling yourself the six untruths listed on page 67, under section 2).

d) Appreciate the friendships and love you do have in your life.

e) If you haven't any friends, learn how to make them. (It's never too late to learn.) When one woman told us she was lonely and asked for our help, we suggested she write down three ways in which she kept other people at a distance. She wrote these, and by being honest, she quickly realized how she was keeping herself lonely. Her list may be something like yours:

- talking constantly about yourself.
- being negative much of the time: "Isn't it awful?" "If it weren't for you"..."What's the matter with Charlie?"
- being a victim ("Poor little me!") and really believing no one else has any real troubles.

To be with this woman was a "downer." People avoided her because she made them feel heavy and burdened. When she was willing to change her self-destructive behavior, she began to make friends.

When we counsel people who say they have no friends, we tell them that since all of us began life as loveable, being friendless now is a result of learning how to keep people away. If friendless people will risk changing their "stay away from me" behavior and begin slowly to trust others, to feel safe around other people, they will soon realize how much most people want closeness and friendship. If they will then be genuinely interested in others and not over-demanding, they will make first one friend, then two or three, and finally a whole circle of real friends. When next you feel lonely, remember what you have done by taking these five steps (described above) to ease your pain, and then do them all over again. Keep at it. It does work.

There is another kind of loneliness often called existential loneliness; that is, loneliness experienced as part of our human condition. Existential loneliness is of an entirely different nature from the one just discussed. Traditional

Jewish and Christian theologians, as well as theologians in
other religious traditions, believe that existential loneliness is what humankind experiences when separated from
God. I came from God, belong now to God, and will at
death return to God; I will then experience loneliness of an
existential kind whenever in this life I separate myself
from God by disobedience, apostasy, or mistaking my ego
for God's will. "That you may be as gods" was the original
biblical temptation in the book of Genesis. To live with
God as the center of the universe and of my own life is to
feel connected, a part of, belonging to, a member of, one
community with those myriad others, past and present,
who also believe God to be Lord, creator, director, the one
from whom we all came, to whom we all now belong, and
to whom we will all return. When, however, I live under
the dominance of my little ego to the detriment of others, I
feel cut off from the Center of life. When I gossip about
others, hurt them by my sarcasm, use them to make myself feel better, keep them down economically so that I may
have more and more while they have less and less, then I
feel lonely. When I pay no attention to their cries for help,
food, clothing, medicine, and a decent standard of living,
then I feel alienated from them. When most of my time,
energy, and money go to surrounding myself with pleasure and comfort at the expense of their well-being, then I
experience alienation. Apartheid, racism, military aggrand-
izement, injustice in housing unemployment, inequality
of economic opportunity all tell the real story of our lack of
love and concern for the poor and needy of our world.
This then is the source of our loneliness as we cut ourselves off from our brothers and sisters in the human family of God. Loneliness of this kind can be healed only by
our giving ourselves for the healing of those who have
been wounded by our selfishness and greed.

There is still another kind of loneliness which, however

strange it may seem, is a gift from God. How, you say, could loneliness ever be viewed as one of God's gifts? St. Augustine, one of the great bishops of the early church, wrote of God, "Thou hast made us for thyself and our hearts are restless until they rest in thee." If we were ever fully satisfied, if we were ever truly content short of living under God, we would then have found some kind of promissory god, a god who promised peace and fulfillment but who could never give what he promised. Throughout history this has been the downfall of leaders from Herod in Jerusalem, Cyrus of Persia, all the Caesars, and the Louises, down to the Hitlers and Stalins of our time. Despite grandiose promises, no earthly war lord can give us peace of soul. The same holds true for the very personal mothers, fathers, husbands, wives, and children in our very personal lives. No matter how close we are to parents, children, or marriage partners, these are not God, and if we project on them the task of curing our loneliness, we burden them far beyond reason. Devotion to the idols on our pedestals often turns to anger, and sometimes hate, when these "gods and godesses" do not bring us what we believed they would bring.

God's gift to us is the gift of which St. Augustine wrote. We were made by God, and until we come to know God as our Lord, the Center of our beings, we will continue to feel out of tune, cut off, bereft, desperate, restless, inert, and very, very lonely. Some of us seem driven to put our faith again and again in demi-gods, but the half-gods fail, and when they are finally abandoned, then God who is truly God comes, and we are willing to know God as God is: our indwelling, our Center, our circumference.

Whenever we come to know the truth of St. Augustine's words late in our lifetime or early, it is then for the first time that we will know we are deeply a part of all humankind, we are part of all other men and women who have lived throughout history and who will live in all to-morrows. It is then that we know God for what God is—our beginning, our reason for being, our final haven from loneliness and death.

What we have said in this chapter will not keep any of us from occasional feelings of loneliness. It will, however, give us an insight into what kind of loneliness we feel and what its source probably is. If we are lonely because of childhood wounds and childhood decisions that "It will always be like this," we can recognize this fact and make a decision to move out of our childhood position of sulk and anger; we can decide to become aware that like all humankind we are fragile, hurt human beings who need very much to love and be loved. If our loneliness is the result of our allowing our selfishness to be the center of our lives and thus cut us off from others by ego-aggrandizement, then we can turn from selfishness to become persons of care and charity toward ourselves and other people. If our loneliness comes from genuine seeking after God, but we have not found God or have found God only tentatively and served God carelessly, then we can take seriously what was spoken to the Israelites: "Hear, O Israel, the Lord your God is one God, and you shall love the Lord your God with all your heart, all your mind and all your soul." Jesus, having been asked to summarize the commandments, placed this first and then said, "The second is like unto it. Thou shall love thy neighbor as thyself." When we learn the truth of obedience to these two commandments, we are one with ourselves, one with our neighbors (all humankind), and one with God.

# Chapter 12

# Families of Choice

Karen had come for her second therapy session. Her flushed face and red eyes gave way to new tears as she talked of being alone. Her children were airplane hours away. Her husband had died some months ago. Now she was one of the seven million women and two million men over the age of sixty who were alone.

Everywhere she turned she saw people belonging to each other in families. She felt lost in a world of people close to one another, having fun, helping, loving. No wonder she cried. Karen had never heard of "families of choice."

We live in a culture in which the importance of the family is emphasized by the media, the church, politicians, and the community. Yet the harsh reality is that many have no family and others have little or no meaningful contact with their families. Thirty percent of the households in the United States are occupied by one person. The percentage of older adults living alone is higher than ever.

These figures are frightening to many people and depressing for others. Some who have spouses live in fear that their spouse will die first and leave them isolated and alone.

Over and over again in their offices and at the workshops they lead, the authors hear statements like, "It's a couples' society," "I can't bear to think about living alone," "No women want widows, divorcees, or single people around when their husbands are there. Sure, they will invite us to eat lunch or to join the women's clubs, but that's all."

Some fortunate people have close families—brothers, sisters, cousins, parents, children, grandchildren, or in-laws who live within visiting distance and who enjoy being together. Some are close in feeling but are separated by distance; some have no families at all; others are separated emotionally to the point where they do not want to be together.

This can be sad and lonely. But people who do not have the sense of family they want do not need to keep the situation that way for the rest of their lives.

There are many ways of thinking about "family." Traditionally and legally a family is a group of two or more people who are related to each other biologically or by marriage. Although customs vary greatly, family also implies loving, a mutual sense of belonging, caring for each other's well being and a sharing of physical and material possessions. In a sense, that is the fact of and the spirit of family.

When it is not possible to have a biological family or when members of biological families decide to enlarge their families, adoptive and contractual families can be viable options.

One of the authors does the home studies for, and works with, families who have applied to adopt children from other countries. Of all the work she has done, this is by far the happiest. Couples who have wanted children for years and have not been able to have them, couples who have children of their own and deeply desire more, and single people who want a child even though they choose not to marry are delighted and deeply thankful for the joy these children bring. Children who go to these homes where they are wanted so much that their parents go to great trouble and expense to get them, are similarly privileged. Parents who are pleased to share their love, lives, and possessions with them provide a sense of security these children have never known.

Parents who have biological as well as adoptive children frequently remark how surprised they were to discover that they feel just as close to and have as much sense of family with the adopted ones as they do with their biological children.

Think about yourself and your family in fact and in spirit. Your family may be just the way you want it to be and you may have no desire or need to add to it in any way. You may have a fine family and room in your heart to invite another to be a brother, a granddaughter, or a cousin.

No matter what the situation is with you and your family, you can, and at some time may, decide you will invite another person to be an "adopted relative." The kind of adoption or contractual agreement we are writing about is not a change of legal status. It is something done voluntarily by two people for their mutual benefit and welfare and which includes as many of the elements of good and healthy family spirit as they choose—loving, a sense of belonging, sharing, and caring. These family-of-choice agreements do not involve rejection or renunciation of other family ties, nor are they sexual.

Since many of our readers may not be familiar with this concept, we will give several examples of people who have developed families of choice. Some of these commitments are lifelong; some are so close they defy the saying "Blood is thicker than water." Others are much more casual. The common and essential elements are that these are voluntary agreements for the benefit of both persons concerned and are harmful to no one. Here are some examples (all names are fictitious):

Billy was fond of his grandmother, who died when he was five. When he was in his twenties and still missed having a grandmother, he and an older friend adopted each other as grandson and grandmother. They visited, exchanged letters, cards and small gifts—and kept each other informed of important events.

Madeline, a woman alone and in her sixties, adopted

Mary, a happily married mother of several children, when she was pregnant with her last child (Mary's mother had died when she was young). They visited, and Madeline helped Mary's family emotionally and financially. Mary baked goodies for Madeline, and when the child was born Madeline adopted her as her grandchild.

Elizabeth and Suzanne adopted each other as sisters over twenty years ago. Both had always wanted a sister. Now they have one in spirit and enjoy sharing all that close biological sisters might do.

# Chapter 13

# Journaling

Carl Jung, the great Swiss psychiatrist, believed that we all have a story inside of us. If we write that story of our journey through life, we will see ourselves and our life in a way not otherwise possible. In Chapter 1, we called this storytelling "life review," and suggested that this review would be a good starting place for those who wanted to age with joy. Now we want to speak about "journaling," something many of you may already be doing and want to continue; something you may want to begin if you have never done it.

A journal is a book in which I write my inner story as it is occurring daily, weekly, monthly. Unlike a diary, it has more than a listing of events which meter my days. It is concerned with the meaning of those events. A way to think about these two levels, event and meaning, is to think about recording a video tape. What is put on video-tape are those words, actions, and happenings that can be seen and heard. Such events may be either mundane or unusual. My words and actions may be simple or compli-cated, but the videotape will record them all.

Paralleling these activities and this flow of words that others may see and hear on the videotape, something else is going on simultaneously, inside of us, and it is as if an-other invisible recorder is playing in our head. In Chapter 7, "Talking to Yourself Is OK," we spoke of voices in our head—the way our Parent talks to our Child, our Child to our Parent, our Adult to our Child and Parent, etc. These voices go on in continual conversation in all of us whether we are aware of it or not. All of this takes place in what we will call the first level of our psyche.

Beneath this first level is a second level, the unconscious, and here too conversations go on endlessly. Carl
Jung believed the personality of each of us has many aspects. He spoke of feminine aspects like "witch," "mother,"
"goddess," "seductress," "earth mother," etc., and mascu-
line aspects like "ogre," "father," "God," "villain," "devil,"
"lover," etc. Each part is in relationship with all the other
parts in our unconscious, and Jung believed we would do
well to become familiar with the many facets of our personality. We all have some notion of these many sides when
we see ourselves act differently in different situations and
when we see others we know do the same. We usually say
of ourselves, "I don't know what got into me" or "I never
knew I was so angry" or "I never knew I could do something like that." We use similar phrases when the behavior
of others shocks or surprises us. "I have no idea why when
he's always so pleasant he would now be so mean." "I can't
understand why when she's always so sweet, she was so sar-
castic to me." Statements like these mean that the unconscious parts of us have slipped through.

Now it is true that many people would rather not know
about these voices in their heads (parent, adult, child) and
probably many more want nothing to do with the unconscious aspects of themselves (witch, lover, trickster, queen,
prince). If one would rather not know, then perhaps it is
possible to live as if these voices and aspects weren't there.
Others become intrigued and excited to know more about
this inner part of themselves. If you are one of these people, a journal may be another door you will want to open.
If you decide to keep a journal, a record of your inner journey, here are some suggestions:

1) Buy a notebook or manuscript book (blank pages bound
together) so that what you are writing is already given the
courtesy of being important. Writing on loose bits of paper
may denote a loose, uncaring attitude toward your writing.

2) Write in your book as often as you want.

3) Date whatever you write.

4) List outward events that may be relevant to the writing. Some examples: moved to a new home, husband sick today, best friend arrived, I should have said "no" to serving on that committee but instead I agreed.

5) Write about your feelings (mad, sad, scared, happy). Put down what you really feel, not what you're supposed to feel or would like to feel. If your feeling is related to a specific person, write a conversation with that person. Be absolutely honest and keep writing just as if you were actually speaking to that person. When you have the answer, write that down too. Stop writing only when the feeling is resolved and you are feeling better (if the original feeling was negative) and happier to have shared it (if it was a good feeling that hadn't been said). If what you are feeling is not related to a specific person, but a group of people or an event, you can dialogue with the group or the event the same way as with a specific person.

Carrying on a conversation is also very helpful to come to know persons in your dreams and how they relate to you, whether they are sinister or benevolent figures.

6) Record your dreams. According to sleep record laboratories, we all dream every night. Some of us remember our dreams easily. Others have difficulty or seem unable to recall dreams. If you want to recall your dreams, the chances are you will find it increasingly easy to do so. Some people keep a small flashlight, paper and pencil by their bedside so that when they awaken in the night or first thing in the morning, they can make a few notes about their dream. Then, when they are able to take time, hopefully soon after waking, they write the dream more fully. It is important in dream recording to write as soon as possible after the dream occurs, so that very little dream content will be lost. The longer the time between dream and writing of the dream,

the more our conscious mind alters the dream.

When we have time to be quiet and reflective, then the dream can be "worked" on. "Worked," with a dream, means finding the meaning or the message the dream wants to convey. "Dreams are the royal road to the unconscious." For those who are willing to travel that road, working with the dream reveals, amplifies, deepens, and enriches our understanding of the dream and its message to us.

7) Active imagination. This is Jung's wording for working with dreams. There are several ways to do this:

a) Dialogue with the person in your dreams as described earlier in this chapter.

b) Write a story to dream the dream onward. This is a story that will start where the dream stopped and will in that sense complete the dream. Don't worry if you think you're making it all up. You are, and in that story you will learn a great deal about yourself which would not otherwise come to consciousness. Never censor what you are writing. Go along, and like the conversation and dialogues of which we spoke, simply let things flow as they will.

c) Write a poem inspired by some aspect of the dream.

d) Select one aspect of the dream that is particularly meaningful to you and which especially draws your interest. Then draw a picture of that aspect. If you are like others, you may feel somewhat foolish and self-conscious about drawing, but remember you are not in an art class. It is your picture of your dream, and if you will draw in a free childlike way, if will be a valuable picture for you. If your journal has small pages, you may want to draw on larger paper and then fold your drawing into your journal, just following the recording of your dream.

e) We also want to mention a form of active imagination even though it cannot be placed in your journal: clay molding and shaping. This can be done with schoolroom clay sold at most art supply stores. Select a figure or simple aspect of your dream and then mold and shape your clay to represent or look like that figure or aspect. Be sure to fire your piece so that it will not break as it dries out. Again, this is a valuable channel through which your unconscious can speak to you.

It's fun to share secrets with friends, and most children like to tease with, "I have a secret and I won't tell." The fun comes in seeing how to get the child to tell, since the decision has already been made that the secret will be told with enough coaxing. But journals are not toys or child games. They are our most private, intimate selves recorded, and as such are best kept to ourselves, shared with no one however intimate, except of course if we are working with a counselor or therapist and this material is part of the counseling session. If any aspect of your journal writing begins to be frightening to you, you have two choices: Stop working with that aspect until a later time when you are feeling more courageous, or find a counsellor trained to accompany you on your inward journey.

One counselee said, "My journal is my best friend. I can tell it anything and it always leads me to know more about myself." May your journal become *your* best friend.

Note: For those interested in a Christian amplification of journal keeping, refer to Morton Kelsey's *Christian Growth Through Personal Journal Writing*, Augsburg Press, Minneapolis, Minn., 1980.

## Chapter 14

# When You Need Help

Let's suppose you have read the earlier chapters of this book, you have followed many of the suggestions, and you are feeling better about yourself. Even so, you are feeling "stuck" about one or more aspects of your life: making new friends, coping with loss, healing a memory, or facing death. Any of these could seem to be "too much"; too bewildering, frightening, or confusing for your to pursue further. If you come to this point, you have three choices: (1) Close the door and decide not to look further at this particular area of your life; (2) close the door for now and decide to look again when you feel stronger; or (3) seek help from a professional counselor or therapist. This chapter suggests how to find professional help.

You may remember a time years ago when doctors were called only for births, devastating illness, and imminent death. Today, prevention is increasingly the focus of modern medicine, and yearly checkups are common practice for those who want to stave off serious illness. So, too, years ago people turned to psychiatrists and mental hospitals when those they loved were obviously disoriented from reality and therefore unable to deal with daily life. Today, most people who seek professional therapeutic help do so to enhance their lives or to obtain help with problems which are unpleasant or uncomfortable for themselves or their families and friends.

If you are considering professional help, you will need to think about two questions: (1) How do I know if I need professional help? (2) If I do think I need it, how do I choose from among the many professionals?

The first question can be answered only by you yourself and the particular counselor you are asking for that help. Here are some guidelines to follow, however:

1) Is the discomfort I feel (sadness, anxiety, fear, helplessness, depression) of long standing, or is it only an occasional discomfort?

2) If it occurs fairly often, am I willing to work with someone else to change it, or do I expect a magic solution from a professional person?

3) Am I doing or thinking of doing any harm to myself or someone else?

4) Am I having physical problems (sleeplessness, high blood pressure, skin rash, gastro-intestinal discomfort, poor appetite, aching, etc.) for which there is no apparent physical cause?

5) Am I having trouble returning to my usual sense of well-being after a tragedy in my life?

6) Do I repeatedly feel left out, unloved, put upon, rejected or misunderstood?

If you answered "yes" to several of the above questions, you probably need to look for a professional counselor. The question then is, who? In small towns the choice is limited. In larger cities the choice can be confusing. Actually, the best way to find a good therapist is through referral by someone you already know and trust, especially if that person has received help from the therapist in question.

Several professional disciplines provide the education and training necessary for certification and (in most states) licensing in the field of therapy. Traditionally, therapists have come from three such groups: physicians, psychologists, and social workers. More recently, some nurses and clergy have taken additional training to become therapists. The number of professional counselors is also growing.

Unfortunately some professional competiveness has manifested itself among these groups. In reality no group is more competent than another; each includes excellent therapists as well as some incompetent practitioners. All have essentially the same training and education in the basic information necessary to become effective therapists: human development, personality theory, healthy vs. pathological thinking, feeling, and behavior, diagnosis of problems, evaluation of strengths, and methods of treatment. In addition to this general body of knowledge, each discipline has its own specialty. Psychologists are experts in psychological testing and diagnosis; psychiatrists have additional training in organic anomalies, pathology and medication, and are authorized to prescribe medication and hospitalization; social workers are experts in dealing with individual problems relating to a person's family and culture.

Still another choice faces you if you are looking for professional help in a well-populated area. Do you want a therapist in private practice or one in a clinic, mental health center, or family service agency? We suggest that you check into the differences in your community between agencies and private therapy, and then evaluate those differences in terms of your reason for wanting help and your expectations for treatment. Here are some suggestions to help you as you make your decision. First the negative suggestions:

1) Don't go to anyone unless you can find at least one other person (beside your doctor) to recommend this therapist.

2) Don't continue to go to anyone who tells you it will take a very long time in treatment before you will be OK. You decide that.

3) Don't keep on with anyone about whom you continue to have bad feelings. Trust your intuition.

4) Don't assume that the higher the academic degree, the better the therapist.

5) Don't assume that the higher the fee, the greater the skill.

6) Don't continue to see a therapist who at your first in-

terview wants to hospitalize you, unless you are highly suicidal, homicidal, chemically addicted, or losing touch with reality. Thousands of people are hospitalized unnecessarily each year because physicians and hospitals gain financial advantages. Be especially careful of institutions that advertise widely, offer free consultations, and are interested primarily in your insurance coverage.

The positive suggestions:

1) Find the best therapist available. You deserve the best.

2) Be open and honest about what you're wanting in therapy. Check out the qualifications, experience, and continuing education of the therapist.

3) Check out cost, method of payment, insurances, length of sessions, cancellation policy, and the expected length of time for fulfilling your needs.

4) Look for the person who is qualified, understanding, and concerned; you must feel a real rapport with your therapist. Trust yourself in this.

5) Evaluate your first appointment in light of the four suggestions above. Make a second appointment only if you feel you will get what you need by working with this therapist. Better to go to another person than put yourself in a losing position.

6) Keep at it. There are painful times in therapy. When therapy is effective, you will feel better about yourself almost from the beginning.

# Chapter 15

# The Final Years

Few of us want to think about the final years of our lives. We want to believe we will live forever. Often this is true even of people whose lives have been difficult or who are in great distress. Despite our strong will to live, we cannot escape the final stages of our lives.

We have identified three stages of aging:
- Early aging: a period of renewed energy
- Middle aging: our world grows smaller
- Elder aging: increased dependency

Many people find it easy to live happily in the years of early aging. This chapter offers help for those in middle and elder aging so that these stages may also have meaning and joy.

Commenting on middle aging, the period from retirement to mid or late seventies, we hear many people say, "I've never had it so good!" Job responsibilities are over and children are grown. For many people this is a time for travel, for studying in adult programs at universities or Elderhostels, for reviewing life, for saying goodbye to self-destructive behavior, and for enjoying what is called "the golden age." If there is no devastating illness during this time, if finances allow us to meet daily expenses and still have something left over for fun and travel, if we have lived our earlier years with a fair degree of insight and honesty, if we love the past, enjoy the present, and are courageous about tomorrow, then this will be a wonderful segment of our life.

This period of the younger aging years comes to a close usually in our late seventies, sometimes in the mid-eighties. We have lived in the ten-to fifteen-year period immediately following our retirement or mid-sixties; now another change takes place. Travel is less frequent, and some of us seem not interested in traveling at all unless it is absolutely essential. We have the feeling of having been everywhere, or if we have never been anywhere we feel that going is just too much effort. Organized activities hold less interest than they did, although we may occasionally be part of a class, club, or activity group. At this time some of us move from our own homes into retirement communities, or into homes of family members, or even into group homes with surrogate families. Our world grows a little smaller.

Given these inner changes of mind and heart which have led to changes in outer activity, the period of the late seventies to late eighties can still be one of rich meaning and joy. Here are some people in this age group with whom we talked for this book:

1) Marvin, age 83, remarried two years ago after being widowed. He rides his bicycle almost daily and adds much to groups by singing his favorite old songs in his lovely tenor voice. Marvin had cancer a couple of years ago, but says he doesn't have time to worry.

2) Magdalene, age 87, walks a mile every day even though her knees hurt. She makes friends instantly with her smile, her sparkling blue eyes, and her stories about early life in Norway.

3) Lee, age 81, teaches creative writing in a continuing education school for adults. She writes every day herself and swims daily for an hour. With her keen mind and interests, she is a challenge for everyone.

4) Tom, age 85, a retired professor, helps anyone interested in landscaping or gardening, and with laughter in his voice, tells stories of early life in Holland and days of settling in this country as a Dutch immigrant.

5) Emily, a watercolor artist, painted until she was 96, walked every day until six months before her death, read avidly, and had almost constant "open house" for her myriad friends and students.

6) Among the famous whose zest for life keeps or kept them growing and giving into their late years are: comedian George Burns; choreographer Agnes de Mille, and Queen Mary of England, mother of the present queen.

What we have just described as a two-stage period may for some be telescoped into one. For some the very fact of retirement or reaching the "golden age" may bring on physical or emotional ill health. Whether we have somehow "brought it on ourselves" or whether it has been visited on us, we are in real pain and suffering. If we are harassed by poor health, money shortage, and mindsets of mistrust, depression and fear, then our final years are moved closer by ten or more. We hope that in this book we have offered thoughts and practical guidelines to help aging people change some of their ways of living so that they can be assured of better health, greater emotional well-being, and deeper spiritual meaning.

Whether the period beyond the sixties is a two-stage period or it is telescoped into one, no matter how many years we live, there comes a time when we have only a few remaining years. We have not yet been told that we are going to die shortly, but we know we have slowed down so much that we are indeed elderly. We have long been acquainted with aches and pains, but now they are worse and irreversible. Eyesight, hearing, mobility, all or one have weakened, and as we need help to move, see, or hear we are thrust further and further into a little world of our own. We can no longer easily get to our friends. Even if we could, many of them may have died long ago. We can no longer take ourselves shopping, or go to a movie, a church supper, a club meeting. Television must be louder for us to hear; we see it less clearly; or if we can hear it quite well perhaps we can no longer see much. Groups make us nervous—they are too stimulating or there is too much noise and conversation.

In this period of our life, we are forced to face ourselves as never before. Some of us may face ourselves for the first time. The escape hatches are closed. We are in a wheelchair, in a room, dependent, seemingly separated from life outside, seemingly useless, and just taking up space, time and money. We dwell more and more on this final condition before our death, and so we become depressed over our boredom, grief, anger, and despair.

If you are living now in the situation we have just described, you may well tell others that they have no real understanding since they do not have the experience with this period of life that you have. You may well reject anything written or suggested because "They have not lived in my shoes." True enough, but if you are willing to keep reading you'll still find some suggestions that may be of help to you.

1) Look again at Chapter 1 and begin your "life review" if you have not done so already.

2) Work at healing your memories so that the painful ones no longer hurt you and the beautiful ones grow like flowers in your memory garden.

3) Find a Listening Partner if you do not already have one. Ask your partner to tell you things that he or she likes about you, not things you accomplish, but you. Do the same for your partner.

4) Read the chapters on pain and loss and begin to practice some of the suggestions in those chapters.

5) Hang on to all five life preservers.

6) Begin to keep a journal or keep on with the one you started.

7) Read again the material on death and dying, and begin

now to make friends with the coming days of death and dying.

If you are unable to do any of the seven things we have just listed, here are five other ways to give each of your days more meaning than they otherwise would have. "Today is the first day of the rest of your life." And so for these last days:

1) Each day focus on one thing you are still able to do and allow yourself to enjoy that one thing, whether it be seeing, hearing, talking, walking, feeding yourself, or getting dressed.

2) Each day focus on one thing you have and allow yourself to enjoy that one thing, whether it be a comfortable bed, enough food, warmth, clothing, a safe place to live, or people to take care of you—family, friends, or nursing home attendants and employees.

3) Focus on a wonderful memory.

4) Give a gift away: a smile, a kind word, a hug, a telephone call to a lonely person.

5) Every day ask for a gift for yourself: someone to hold your hand, rub your shoulders, read to you, or move you to a window or outside.

Those of us who are caring and compassionate would wish that none of us grow old and sick and spend these last days separated from loved ones. In our modern society, however, this seems not to be possible. We have prolonged life by many years, and by so doing we may have prolonged suffering for some. We hope that in these your final years what we have written may ease your burden and heal many of your wounds, so that when the final moments of death and dying come to you, you have courage to endure what you must, thankfulness for the joy you have had in life, and eager anticipation of the life that is to come.

# Chapter 16

# Coping With Death

Why is it that the thought of death brings a shudder to so many of us? We don't even want to think about death— our own or that of our loved ones. But fear that is faced is fear that is lessened. Let us face our fear together.

Even our nation does not want to think about death. We are a young nation that has only recently moved from childhood to adolescence, and we are still enamored of how clever we are to put men into space, turn silicone chips into billion dollar businesses, and put artificial hearts into the dying. Years ago a death was a community experience in the same way that birth and marriage were. When a person died, the community mourned. The body was viewed at a wake; men, women, and children wept. Churches were the place of funeral services. Mourners went to the graveside and saw the deceased person lowered into the ground: "Ashes to ashes, dust to dust." A wreath was placed on the door of the bereaved family. Mourning clothes were worn for an appropriate time by those closest to the dead person. Every one knew that Charles or Marion was really dead.

Today, cremations are more and more frequent. People "pass on" or are "lost." Memorial services are held without bodies, and the community barely notices the death.

This change may at first sight appear to be the result of healthier attitudes toward death than those of our ancestors, but it is more likely that our short shrift practices expose not health but discomfort and unwillingness to face death and dying. But death and dying are real and are one of the common denominators linking all people together.

We all must face death in two forms: our own, and the death of those we know. It is often easier to cope with the first, but we would like to begin this chapter by exploring how to cope with the death of others.

It is a painful fact that the closer we are to another person, the more difficult it is for us to cope with their dying. So much has been unsaid, so much undone; so many memories, so great a loss. There are some things, however, that will enable us to bear the loss of a loved one more adequately. Dr. Kubler Ross has probably studied and researched death and dying more than any other person in modern times. Her books are especially helpful for those trying to bear the burdens and reality of the death of loved ones. As we face such death, almost all of us seem to experience several similar feelings in similar situations. If we know this it may be easier for us to own our own feelings.

1) Denial: "He or she is not going to die." "He or she is not really dead (sleeping, unable to communicate, but not really dead.)"

2) Anger: "Why did it happen?" "God really let me down." "I hate everyone." "They let me down."

3) Sadness: "Will I be able to live without him (or her)?"

4) Fear: "I'm afraid to be alone." "I'll never again have anyone who loves me."

5) Guilt: "If only I had done more for...." "If only I had called the doctor sooner." "If only I hadn't been so unkind."

It is very important for us to be aware of these feelings when they arise and to know that each may arise several times as we are coping with death. The crucial thing is to allow each feeling to go to its full depth and then to face its ramifications consciously, whatever they may be. In Chapter 5 we outlined several ways to relate to our own feelings. In dealing with the death of others, such exploration and expression can bring us much needed healing.

When it is time and we are healed enough, then we must begin life anew. The deeper the pain, the longer time for healing—but life must go on. It is possible to begin again while at the same time carrying a feeling of loss. A year is a realistic period of time for grief over a close friend or loved one. Grief carried beyond that period, grief which debilitates us and keeps us from renewed life, is grief for which we should ask professional help from the clergy, a counselor or therapist. They will help us with what is called grief work so that we can go beyond death to life.

The practical aspects of dealing with death, such as funeral details, legal matters, housing needs, etc., have been written about extensively in other books and articles. Our concern here is to talk about feelings relating to the death of those we love.

We face the issue of death not only as we live through the death of others, but inescapably as we face the matter of our own death. This reality usually has two aspects, a "now" and a "then." The "now" aspect means that right now I must realize that in some tomorrow I, like everyone else, will die. No one lives forever, and no matter what my life has been it will some day come to an end in space and time. The sooner I can say, "I will die in some tomorrow," the sooner I will be able to accept that reality and begin to live with the knowledge as to what that means.

As we have talked with people who have been close to death, and who have gone on living, they all tell us that facing their own death was for them the beginning of living a deeper and more meaningful life. Does the facing of death make life seem more precious? Monks of the Middle Ages kept a human skull on their desks below which were the words, "Remember, O man, thou art but dust." Some people would say that such a practice was morbid. Others might say that such a practice keeps life in perspective and heightens one's appreciation of living.

Once we have accepted the reality of our own death, it is easier to face it when it is imminent. Many people have sudden deaths from heart attacks, car accidents, and acute diseases. Most of us, however, are given warnings of death. How do we cope? Here are some suggestions:

1) Review the five feelings we spoke of when coping with the death of others. These same feelings come again and again as we face our own dying; they need to be allowed their full depth and exploration whatever the consequences.

2) A life review as outlined in Chapter 1 can be begun if it has not already been started. If it has been written earlier, it can now be reread, relived, and reloved.

3) The healing of memories can also be started and if already worked through can be reviewed and added to.

4) Your listening partner may need to be changed or another added, if your chosen listening partner is uncomfortable with death or not available as often as you need to talk.

5) Review the material in chapters six through nine and then look at chapters twelve and thirteen, reading with new eyes and hearing with more sensitive inner ears.

6) Trust that you have done and been enough and that as your physical body weakens, dies, and returns to dust, the essence that is you will live more and more in the light that is to come.

Every dark, painful, agonizing experience of our lives is a part of the whole. We would not be able to have the gift of light if we did not have the gift of darkness. It is difficult to realize this wholeness when we are coping with death, but many philosophers and theologians assure us that dark and light are alike and that we cannot really know life until we have encountered death. Here, as in other pain, we can know that out of death life will come again.

# Chapter 17

# God's Business

"For heaven's sake, what on earth is God doing?" God is doing God's own work: creating, making all things beautiful, loving creation. If this is God's business, for heaven's sake, what on earth are we supposed to be doing?

Since we are made in the image of God, we are to do what God does. We are to create, make our creations beautiful, and love what we create. Creation for us can be making a beautiful home, creating a beautiful child, composing a piece of music, developing a good idea, setting a table, repairing an automobile, making love. Whatever it is we create, if it is beautiful and done in love, it is your business and God's business.

We have really been talking about God's business in our entire book, for God is present in all life, in all growth, and in all healing. He is the creator of all life, the enabler of growth and healing. In this chapter we want to focus more specifically on what is theologically called eschatology, a term derived from Greek, meaning "last things." As the curtain once rose on the beginning of life, so it will one day descend. Eschatology concerns the end of all life, the end of all time. It is difficult for humans to talk of "before" time, a time when there was no time. It is almost impossible to grasp what that would mean. Equally difficult is to imagine a moment when time is no more and the curtain falls. But theologians and ordinary men and women can grasp the idea of beginning and end. The beginning and end are matters of cosmic creation and eschatology. Eschatology also has a personal meaning for each of us—the question asked from the beginning of human history: "What happens when I die?"

If we ask again, "For heaven's sake, what on earth is God doing?" and we answer in terms of creation, this then has everything to do with how we see our own death. You and I need to remember that if we have spent time and effort to make a beautiful object, such as a picture, a poem, some embroidery, a piece of woodworking, or a lovely garden, we would not think of purposely destroying what we have made. So too God would not destroy creation, of which we humans are a valuable part. The potter takes clay, molds it, shapes it, and fires it in the kiln. At each step, the clay changes form and becomes more beautiful, and in its final form it will last for many years. So in each stage of our life we are molded and shaped and finally undergo the firing of death; but faith teaches us that we are not thereby destroyed, and that we will in some way live forever. St. Paul talks about an earthly body that is seen, touched, and felt, but after death is no longer needed. He then tells us of a celestial, heavenly body that cannot be seen with earthly vision, but is nonetheless real. The book of Revelation in the Bible talks of last things by saying that in life after death there shall be no night and that God will wipe away all tears. This is poetical or symbolic language for speaking about the passing away of pain, sorrow, anguish, and heartbreak. Jesus tells us that he has come that we might have life and have it abundantly, that he is the resurrection and the life, and that whosoever believes in him shall never die, but have everlasting life.

Of course, some men and women tell us that when we die we end all life, that there is nothing more, that all statements of life beyond death are made by wishful thinkers who are weak and fear death's final victory. Others say, "Prove life after death and I'll believe." Still others say they are not concerned with what, if anything, happens on the other side of death.

Truth, it may be said, "is in the eyes of the beholder,"

and there is nothing we can say to someone who finds belief in life after death unnecessary, irrelevant, incomprehensible, or a matter of wishful thinking.

For those with faith, such a belief is none of these things. It is a clear promise that in God's business, everything is created from divine love and made in beauty. "A thing of beauty is a joy forever."

"And God shall wipe away all tears from their eyes and there shall be no more death, neither sorrow nor crying, neither shall there be anymore pain; for the former things are passed away. There shall be no night there and they need no candle, nor the light of the sun, for the Lord God giveth them light. (Revelation 21:4)

"I am the Alpha and the Omega, the beginning and the end." (Revelation 22:5)

We are God's creation, made beautifully in the divine image. We will live with God forever and ever. We can age with joy!

# APPENDIX A

## RESOURCES FOR SENIORS AND
## THOSE WITH AGING OR AILING LOVED ONES

*Aging Network Services* (ANS) A private service specifically designed to address problems confronting adult children with aging parents living in other areas. ANS provides a comprehensive and preventative plan designed to maintain independence to the greatest extent for aging loved ones while providing peace of mind to concerned adult children. ANS works with a nationwide network of qualified clinical social workers who assess the parent's condition and arrange for necessary services. Barbara Kane (301) 986-1608 or Grace Lebow (301) 951-8589 will provide a free half-hour consultation to introduce the service to you.

*Alzheimer's Family Support Groups* "A Manual for Group Facilitators" is available at U.S.F. Suncoast Gerentology Center, University of Southern Florida, Box 50, 12901 N. 30th Street, Tampa, Fl. 33612.

*American Association of Retired People* (AARP) 1909 K Street NW, Washington. D.C. 20049. A 20 million person organization which provides information, service and money savers to those over 50. Programs and services include advocacy, consumer education, community programs, health, learning opportunities, media resources, research, volunteer pursuits, etc. To join, send $5.00 to AARP, P.O. Box 199, Long Beach, Cailf. 90801.

*American Bar Association* Commission on Legal Problems of the Elderly, 1800 M Street NW, Washington, D.C. 20036. Provides referrals to competent attorneys. Ask for their free booklet "Doing Well by Doing Good."

*Area Agencies on Aging* State and local agencies are set up under the Older Americans Act. They provide services from counseling to transportation, from legal aid to Meals on Wheels. Look under Social Service Agencies in the Yellow Pages.

*Blue Cross, General Health Insurance* Publishes a directory of physicians by specialty and county, who will accept assignment of

Medicare payments, then bill patients for the twenty percent co-payment.

*Caregivers Inc.* 571 Dauphin St., Mobile, Al. 36603, (205) 433-3206 fosters community awareness, locates lonely, frail, isolated, elderly, or disabled people and their caregivers, recruits volunteers who offer home care, and gives other assistance to the elderly and their caregivers.

*Caring for Dependent Parents* The Research Institute of America, Inc. 589 Fifth Avenue, New York, N.Y. 10017. Provides guidance on how to be well informed and prepared for what the future may hold for you and your elderly parents. $3.95 plus postage.

*Children of Aging Parents* 2761 Trenton Road, Levittown, PA 19056. How to find or start a support group. Good information for caregivers. Membership $10.00.

*Choosing an HMO; An Evaluation Checklist* Provides specific guidelines for older persons who are considering joining an HMO. Free booklet, write AARP Fulfillment, D12444, P. 0. Box 2400, Long Beach, Cailf. 90801.

*Directory of Respite Care Services* 1500 Pelham Parkway, Bronx, N.Y. 10461, (212) 824-4004.

*Eye Care for those over 65* Call 1-(800) 222 EYES. Eligible callers will be mailed the name of a volunteer physician in their area who will treat them regardless of ability to pay.

*Family Caregivers of the Aging* A program of the National Council on Aging. Information and guidance are provided on choosing alternative housing, locating in-home care providers and support groups, understanding Medicare and Medicaid, and legal and financial planning. $25.00 annual membership provides free information, newsletters, and legislative advocacy. The National Council on Aging Inc., 600 Maryland Ave. S.W., West Wing 100, Washington, D.C. 20024.

*Family Service of America* 44 E 23rd Street, New York, N.Y. 10010. Provides direct services or makes referrals for the elderly. Operates in most states.

*Friends and Relatives of Institutionalized Aged Inc.* 425 East 25th Street, New York, N.Y. 10010. Send a stamped envelope for a checklist of nursing homes.

*National Association for Home Care* 519 C Street NE, Stanton, Pk, Washington, D.C. 20002, (202) 547-7424. Home health care referrals, listings of hospital and hospice based services and agencies certified by Medicare.

*National Council on Aging, Inc.* 600 Maryland Avenue SW, West Wing 100, Washington, D.C. 20205. Provides health care information.

*National Home-Caring Council* 235 Park Avenue, New York, N.Y. 10003. Send $2.00 plus self-addressed business envelope with postage for their booklet on how to find the best home care help.

*National Hospice Organization* 1901 N. Fort Myer Drive, Arlington, VA 22209, (703) 243-5900. Information on Hospice care.

*National Institute on Adult Day Care* 600 Maryland Avenue SW, West Wing 100, Washington, D.C. 20024. Referrals in various locations.

*Telephone Silver Pages* Lists business, professional, and service providers who give discounts to senior citizens.

*Telephone Yellow Pages* Look for listings under Aging, Home Health Care, Medical Aids, Nursing Homes, Social Service Agencies, and Senior Citizens.

*Variety of Travel Discounts.* Many airlines give special senior discounts. For the frequent traveler (nine or more trips per year) the best buys are with TWA and Eastern Airlines. Both provide annual fares for virtually unlimited mileage. Participants must be 65 for TWA or 62 or over with Eastern. Both airlines also have companion passes available for a younger companion. Passes run about $1200-1300 per year, there are often specials available also. Eastern and Delta sell packets of 4 or 8 tickets for a flat fee of around $350 and $600 respectively. Braniff offers 5% discount on all tickets for seniors and companions. United and TWA offer 10% for seniors who enroll for a small fee. Call your local carriers or check with your travel agents. Trains, busses and rapid transit authorities frequently have reduced fares, e.g., the Boston Metro system has a flat 10¢ fare for seniors. Always check when traveling.

Hotels and Motels have a variety of discounts. Some require membership in AARP or travel clubs, others do not. Inquire when reserving. Entertainment, from movies to opera and museums, often has special prices. Once again, ask.

Restaurants were among the pioneers in senior discounts. Some highlight their special prices, others require that you ask.

# APPENDIX B

## WHAT OTHERS SAY

A brief questionnaire was sent to various people who appeared to be aging with joy. Here is a summary of their replies. The most frequent answers are listed first.

1) What has been the most helpful thing in your development after age 40?

    Self-acceptance
    Continued study and mental activity
    Loving and supportive family
    Self-insight
    Therapy
    Career change
    Courage
    Curiosity
    Quitting smoking
    The arts

2) What has been the most helpful thing in your development since age 60?

    Continuing to be active—in profession, hobbies, or learning
    Listening and being open to self and others
    Helping others

Accepting or trusting self
Accepting changes
Becoming closer to children
Belief in an afterlife
Good nutrition or exercise
Health
Humor, curiosity, wonder, interests
Enough money not to have to worry
Deeper understanding of the rhythms of life

3) What counsel do you have for others?
Keep active
Stay involved with others and community
Challenge yourself
Keep learning
Appreciate - literature, art, theater, people
Learn to live fully now; use all you have to the hilt
Be good to other people
Build and nurture relationships
Be good to yourself
Be conscious of your body and its needs, including exercise,
    diet, vitamins, and rest
Count your blessings
Love yourself, neighbor, and God
Love life and have awe and reverence for all creation
Travel
Look forward and upward
Laugh often—especially at yourself
Have courage to be different, even eccentric
Accept responsibility—what happens to you is less impor-
    tant than what you do about it
Enjoy doing less—there are great joys available in retirement.

# Appendix C

## "Second Wind Generation"
## If you want to help—

1) Caroline Bird, in her book *The Good Years*, lists five areas that she believes need "pioneers of the 21st century":

   a) Systems patching. As technology breaks down, people are needed to patch it up. As social systems have less government money, more of us are needed as volunteers in schools, social agencies, hospitals.

   b) Conservation. We complain about pollution and poisoning from our environment. We can work for clean air and unpoisoned food.

   c) Experience sharing. We have years of living, wisdom and experience to share. We can find ways to pass it on to those younger.

   d) Matchmaking. We can put together people with ideas, institutions, and others to make a good match.

   e) Whistle blowing. On public officials, bad legislation etc. We have nothing to lose. Let's work for accountability and integrity.

2) In Texas, a group of retired Southern Baptists crisscross the country in motor homes ten months of the year to build rural churches without pay. They have fun. Churches get homes.

3) In California, the "Senior Gleaners" harvest the left-over crops to distribute to the poor.